FUELED

7 PILLARS OF OPTIMAL WELLNESS

A Proven Blueprint for Restoring Health...
God's Way

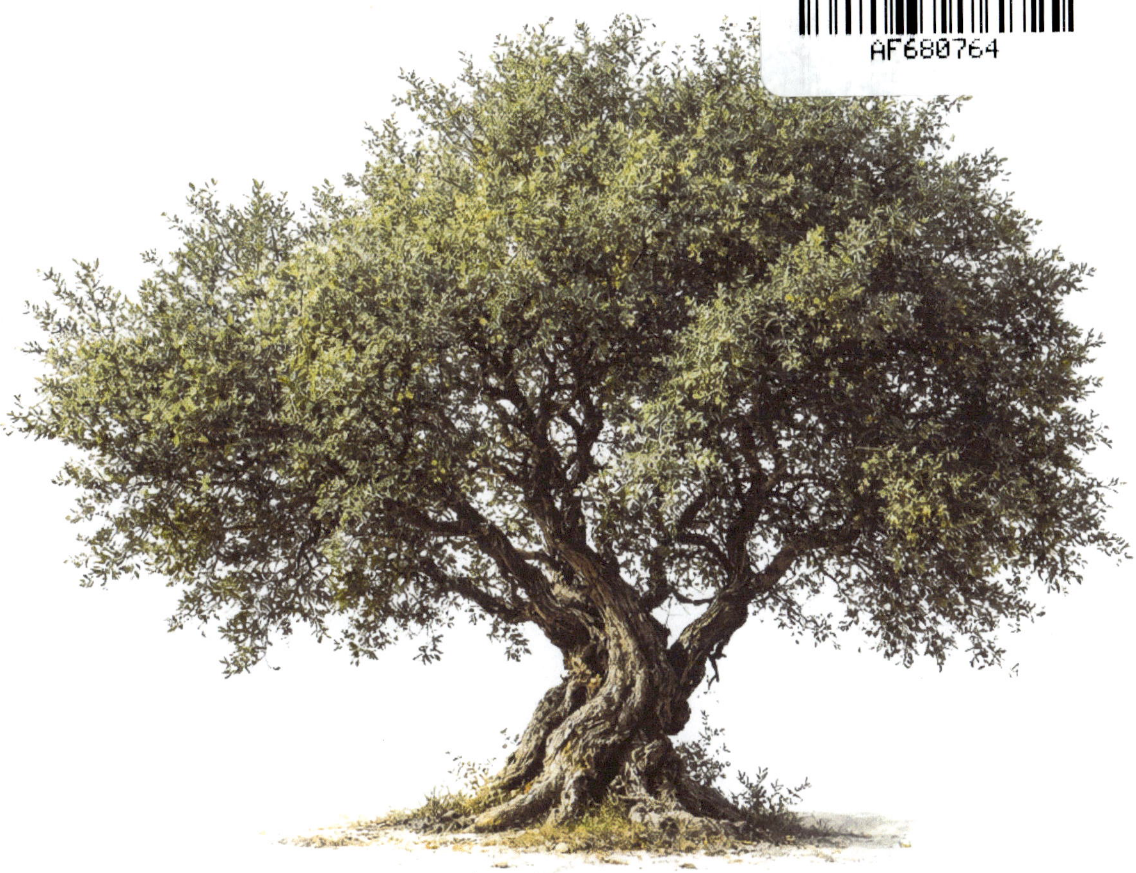

STACI WALLACE

WITH IRINA CHIFOR

Reader Note: Scripture quotations in this work are taken from various Bible translations, including primarily the New International Version (NIV).

Published by Game Changer Publishing

Book Cover and Illustrations by Staci Wallace
www.StaciWallace.com

First edition 2026

Paperback ISBN: 978-1-7327916-7-1
Hardcover ISBN: 978-1-7327916-8-8
Digital ISBN: 979-8-90158-160-5

ACKNOWLEDGMENTS

To my dear family and faithful Fueled by Fire Community for being the proving ground of these life-changing principles for nearly three decades.

Thank you for being God-fearing leaders worth following.

You are here to bring out the God-colors in this world.
Live as an example of the Kingdom of God on earth as it is in heaven.

This is YOUR moment!

Shine.

TABLE OF CONTENTS

> *"For while bodily training is of some value, godliness has value in every way, holding promise for the present life and also for the life to come."*
> **— 1 Timothy 4:8**

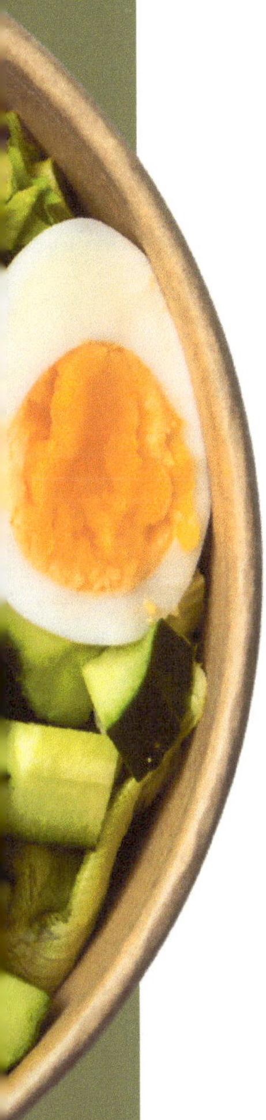

PREFACE

By Irina Chifor, DipION, mBANT, rCNHC

I never planned on becoming a Registered Nutritional Therapy Practitioner or dedicating my life to the study of functional medicine and the root causes of illness. In fact, as a young girl, I dreamed of becoming a ballerina.

But God had a different plan.

My journey began in a hospital room, watching doctors fight to bring my newborn daughter back to life.

Maya was only three weeks old when she went into cardiac arrest. For 45 minutes, doctors worked desperately to revive her. The outlook was grim. The medical team quietly prepared me for the possibility that my baby might not survive.

In the middle of the chaos, surrounded by machines, alarms, and rushing doctors, I did the only thing I knew to do.

I prayed.

Out loud, with every ounce of faith I had, I declared over my daughter,

"Maya, you shall live and not die in Jesus' name."

Against the odds, Maya survived.

But the news that followed was devastating. Doctors explained that the prolonged cardiac arrest had caused significant brain damage. Maya was later diagnosed with quadriplegic cerebral palsy, and I was told she would likely never walk or speak.

What followed was a journey no parent is prepared for. Hospital visits. Specialists. Medications. Protocols. Questions that often led to more questions.

At one point, Maya was prescribed nine different medications and was experiencing frequent seizures, sometimes as many as twenty an hour. Each appointment seemed to add another layer of management, yet something in my spirit remained unsettled.

I began asking deeper questions.

What was each medication truly addressing?
What were the side effects?
And was this approach restoring my daughter's health, or simply managing symptoms?

The answers were not always clear.

So I began researching for myself. I studied the medications, their interactions, and the long-term impact they could have on her developing body. My conversations with doctors became more direct, more intentional, and more informed.

In partnership with medical professionals, and through careful, informed decisions, we began reducing what no longer aligned.

Slowly, something remarkable began to happen.

Maya went from nine medications to just one. The seizures that once defined her condition stopped completely. Doctors had said it would not happen.

I do not take credit for that outcome but I recognize God's hand in the decisions that were made. During that season, I spent weeks taking communion nightly beside my daughter's bed, praying and believing for healing and wisdom.

That experience marked a turning point in my life.

It revealed something I could no longer ignore. While medicine plays a vital and life- saving role, it does not always provide all the answers. There are times when healing requires looking deeper, asking better questions, and supporting the body in ways that align with God's original design.

This realization ignited a passion in me to understand the body more fully.

Not long after, my second child began experiencing allergies, digestive issues, and respiratory challenges. Once again, I found myself searching for answers that went beyond symptom management. Through changes in nutrition, gut health support, and a focus on strengthening the body's foundational systems, my son's health began to improve and today he is thriving.

Another defining moment came during my pregnancy with twins.

Classified as high-risk, I was closely monitored throughout the pregnancy. When concerns arose, I chose to support my body through a food-first approach, applying the nutritional principles I had been studying daily.

The results surprised even my medical team. I carried my twins to full term, and my obstetrician spent significant time asking about the nutritional strategies I had used.

These experiences confirmed a pattern I could no longer ignore. When the body is supported properly, it has an extraordinary capacity for resilience and restoration.

With that conviction, I made a life-changing decision. While raising young children, I returned to study nutritional therapy, training at the Institute for Optimum Nutrition in London, one of Europe's leading institutions in functional and personalized nutrition.

Today, I work as a nutritional therapy practitioner, helping people identify root causes, restore energy, rebalance their bodies, and build sustainable habits that support long-term wellness.

But my approach goes beyond physical health. I believe that true wellness involves the alignment of spirit, soul, and body. Lasting transformation happens when faith, mindset, and physical health come into agreement.

As my journey unfolded, I realized that what began as a search for answers for my own family had become something much greater. It had become a calling.

That calling eventually led me to Fueled by Fire. I first came through the Fueled training and certification as a client, seeking to expand my clinical practice from a one-on-one model to a one-to-many practice. What God was actually doing was creating an alignment that would precede a lifelong assignment with Fueled.

When Staci invited me to contribute to this work, it felt like a natural extension of that calling. What began as a personal journey has now become a shared mission to help others restore their health, renew their energy, and live fully aligned with God's design.

In recent years, research has continued to confirm what many of us have been witnessing for a long time. Industrialized food production, highly processed foods, excessive sugars, chemical additives, and nutrient-depleted diets have taken a significant toll on human health.

Many people today are living with digestive issues, poor gut health, weakened immune systems, brain fog, headaches, chronic fatigue, joint pain, and hormonal imbalance. Many are managing symptoms but never addressing the root cause.

This book was written to point toward answers. Toward root causes. Toward solutions that are not new, but ancient—principles that have supported human health for thousands of years and align with how God designed the body to function, heal, and restore.

For more than two decades, Staci Wallace has trained people to transform their lives from the inside out, helping leaders lose hundreds of pounds, restore energy, repair years of neglect, and rebuild their lives with discipline, purpose, and health.

Together, our prayer is that we make simple what often feels complex—the human body as God designed it, and how to use the 7 Pillars to regain, repair, and rebuild a life of optimal wellness.

You were not called to manage symptoms. You were called to thrive.

Here's to living life God's way.

THE SEVEN PILLARS
OF OPTIMAL WELLNESS

When these foundational pillars are fully rooted, the body naturally begins to function the way it was designed.

1. **SPIRITUAL FITNESS**
2. **MENTAL MASTERY**
3. **HYDRATION**
4. **NUTRITION**
5. **MOVEMENT**
6. **REST**
7. **THE JESUS WAY**

HOW TO USE THIS BOOK

This book is not meant to be read once and placed on a shelf. It is a blueprint. Each pillar builds upon the one before it. As you move through the chapters, take time to complete the exercises, reflect on the questions, and allow the Holy Spirit to guide your transformation.

Strong roots produce healthy lives. Let's begin.

PART ONE:
THE RESET

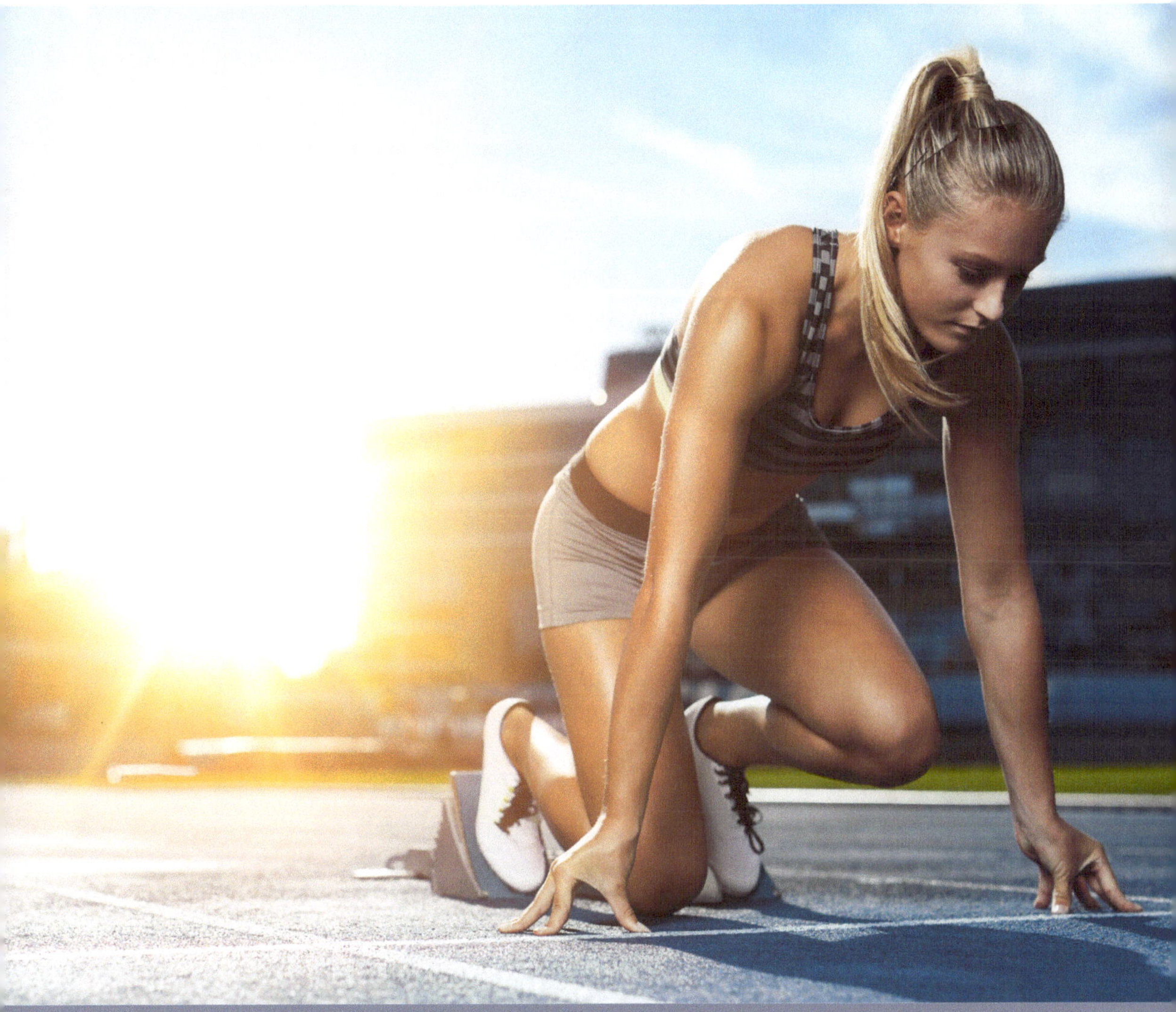

NOT MEDICAL ADVICE
This book is not intended to provide medical advice. As with any changes to diet, nutrition, or fasting practices, consult your healthcare professional before making adjustments to your routine.

Wellness is more than food and exercise.
It is the result of a life aligned with God, where the spirit leads,
the mind is renewed, and the body thrives.

INTRODUCTION

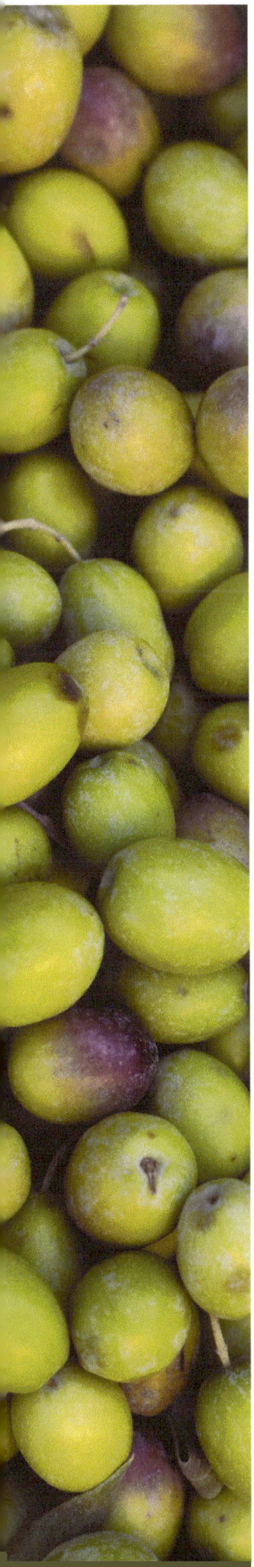

"I have to admit something right from the beginning. I love olives. I love olive oil. I love olive trees. If you spend any time with me in the kitchen, you will quickly discover that olive oil finds its way onto just about everything."

I am not entirely sure when my fascination with olives began. Somewhere along the way, they captured my imagination. Perhaps it was their rich flavor. Perhaps it was their connection to Scripture. Or perhaps it was the quiet strength or silvery leaves of the trees themselves.

When Larry and I moved to Epiphany Ranch and began planting our orchard, I imagined rows of grapevines and olive trees stretching across the hills. In my mind, I could already see the silvery leaves of olive branches dancing in the Texas sun and bottles of our own olive oil sitting on the kitchen counter."

But East Texas had other plans.

Our February ice storms quickly taught me that olive trees do not thrive easily here. My first three attempts ended the same way. The freezing winds won.

Eventually, I realized that if I wanted olive trees at the ranch, they would need to live indoors. Today, my precious potted olive babies sit happily inside Epiphany Lodge, where they are safe from the winter cold.

When it came time to design the cover for this book, we explored many possibilities. Different concepts. Different images. Different directions. Then one day it became obvious. The olive tree is the perfect representation of everything this book stands for.

Throughout Scripture, the olive tree is a symbol of flourishing, covenant, and blessing. In Psalm 52:8, David writes, "But I am like an olive tree flourishing in the house of God; I trust in God's unfailing love forever and ever."

That verse captured my attention because it reveals something profound. Flourishing is never accidental. It is the result of being rooted in the right place and nourished according to the right design.

Olive trees are among the most resilient trees on earth. Some have lived for hundreds, even thousands, of years. They survive drought, intense heat, stubborn, rocky soil, and harsh environments, yet continue to produce fruit generation after generation.

But there is something even more fascinating about the olive tree.

An olive tree thrives when three things are aligned.

Its roots.
Its environment.
Its nourishment.

When those three elements are in harmony, the tree flourishes. In fact, olive trees often produce their richest fruit after seasons of pruning.

And that, my friend, is exactly where this book begins. You are about to step into a journey of restoration, renewal, and rediscovery of how the body was designed to live.

For centuries, these remarkable trees have stood across the hills of Israel and throughout the Mediterranean region. Their twisted trunks tell stories of storms survived, drought endured, and seasons of pruning that ultimately produced richer fruit and greater harvest.

Yet despite their weathered appearance, olive trees remain incredibly productive. Some continue bearing fruit even when they are hundreds of years old.

Scripture often uses the olive tree as a picture of a flourishing life.

A life rooted in God.
A life nourished according to His design.
A life that bears fruit season after season.

The same principle applies to our health.

When our lives are rooted in God's design and nourished according to His blueprint, the body begins to do what it was created to do.

Restore.
Renew.
Strengthen.
Thrive.

The seven pillars you will discover in this book function much like the conditions that allow an olive tree to flourish.

When the roots are strong and the environment is right, the fruit naturally follows. That is the message of Fueled.

True wellness is not something we chase.

It is something we return to.

Let the journey begin!

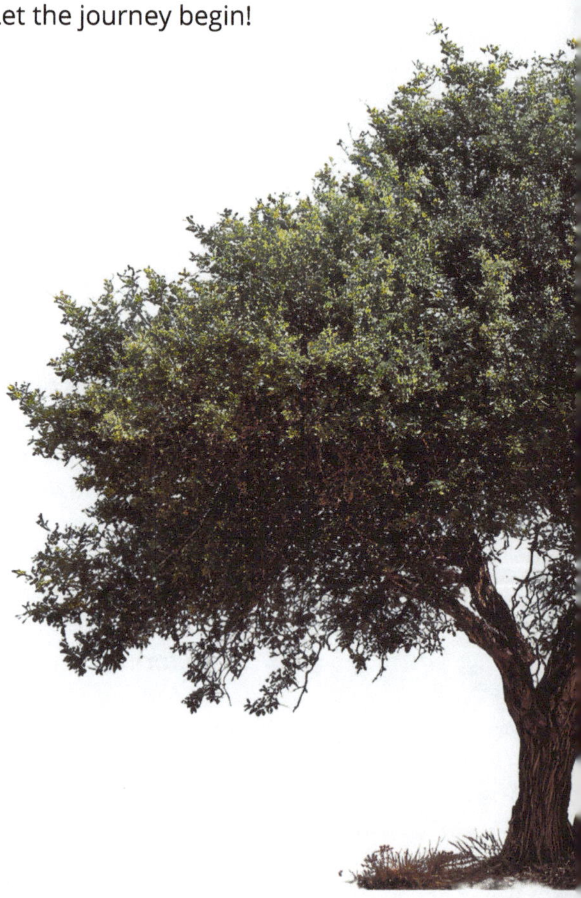

THE OLIVE TREE BLUEPRINT

THE 7 PILLARS OF OPTIMAL WELLNESS

True wellness grows the same way an olive tree grows. Strong roots produce a healthy trunk, and a healthy trunk produces abundant fruit. When the roots are weak, the fruit suffers.

The seven pillars in this book follow that same pattern. First, we strengthen the roots. Then we nourish the body. Finally, we cultivate a life that produces fruit. Flourishing does not happen overnight. It takes time.

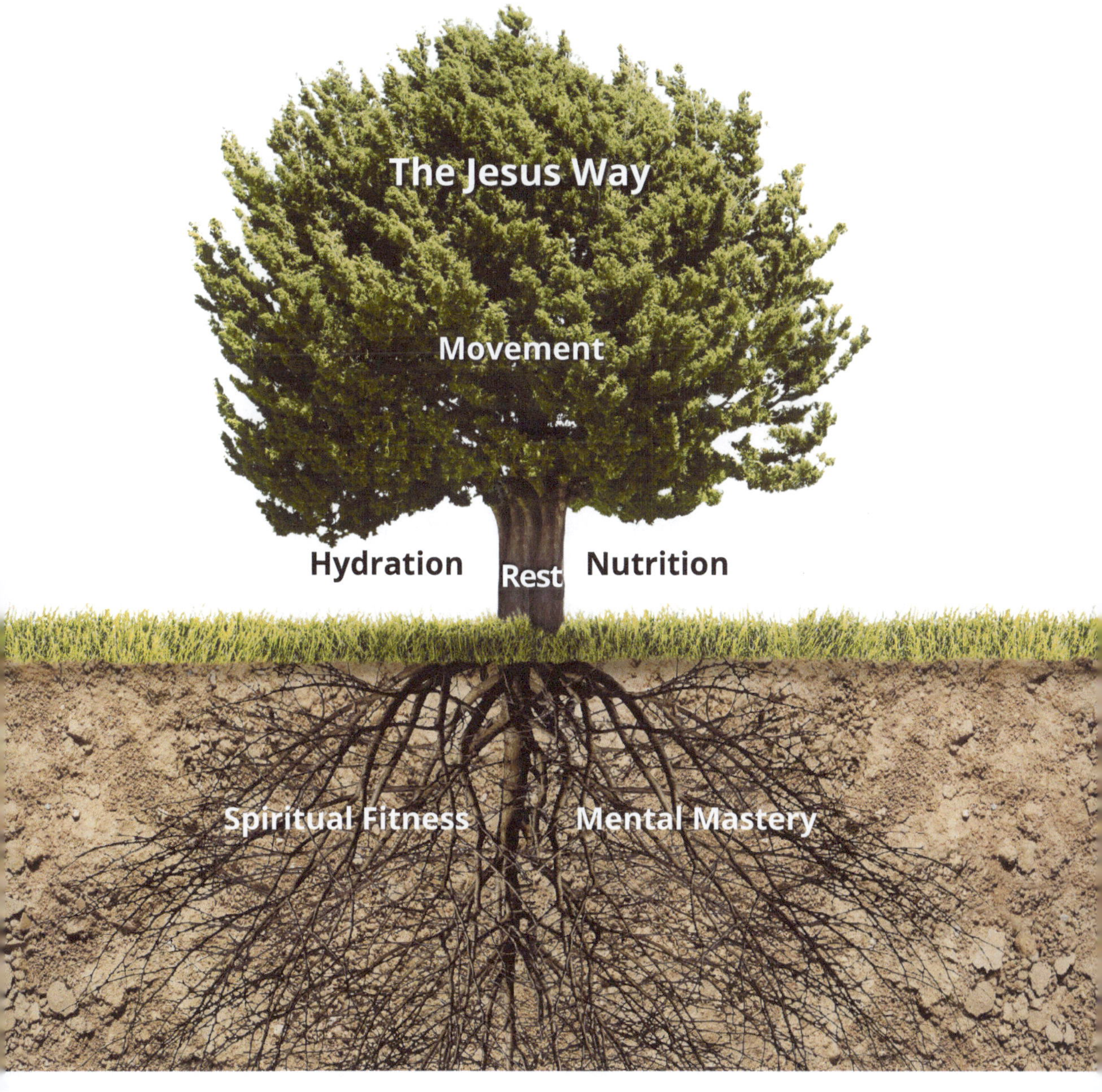

In the chapters ahead, we will strengthen each part of this tree.

SEASONS CHANGE

Looking in the mirror one day, I saw the woman I had promised myself I would never become. When I was twenty-five and in my prime, two women once told me, “Honey, when I was your age, I looked like you, too. Just wait. Time is a kicker.”

I remember thinking they had no idea who they were talking to. I was disciplined. Athletic. Determined. I would never end up like that.

Life, however, has a way of humbling our confidence.

Suddenly, I could relate to the very women I swore I would never become.

As time passed, I moved from my eager twenties and graduated into my birthing thirties, ready to conquer motherhood. I was still rocking along in my 115-pound body, full of energy, pregnant with my first child, and a black belt in karate!

My tight little tushie wasn’t going anywhere, and I was convinced that I would beat the odds of aging, weight gain, and fatigue. Again, I looked at the other mothers around me and vowed that I WOULD NEVER let myself become “like them.”

Larry and I worked out five times per week and played league basketball weekly, further proving that we were never going to change our youthful spirits and bodies.

After our first child, I bounced quickly back into shape. Nursing seemed to strip away the extra baby fat I gained during my pregnancy, and I thought to myself, “That was easy. I could have seven more!” My breasts were perky, and I thought to myself, “Life is great. What’s the big deal? Why do so many women complain? This is easy.”

Then, three months after my first child, I returned to karate. I remember trying to kick that boxing bag with my legs, and it felt like jelly flapping in the wind. I had no muscle control. I thought, “What in the world happened to my lower body? Who cut the cord to my muscles?”

Then I remembered, “Oh yeah... I just gave birth to a 7.5-pound watermelon out of a canal smaller than a quarter! Was it any wonder I might be a tad bit weaker than my pre-baby self?

I refused to accept that my body was changing. Instead, I just decided that high kicks to the head were highly overrated, and so I adopted a killer shin kick and pushed myself back into training to get back to the way things were in my “size 2” days.

With deep resolve, I was absolutely confident that I would NEVER become like “those other mothers with a laundry list of excuses.”

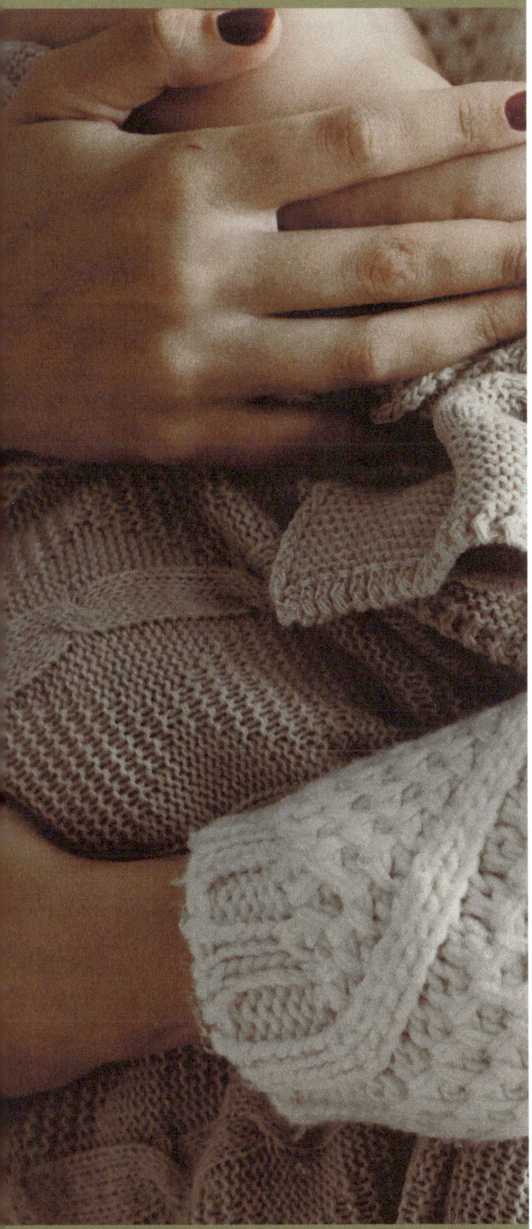

"The stretch marks of our past are the laugh lines of our future. Every scar, every mark is a story of how God gives us the capacity to carry Heaven on Earth in temples made of clay."
— Staci Wallace

"CHANGE IS INEVITABLE"

Then, sixteen months later, I gave birth to our precious baby girl. When I was pregnant with her, my body went through some kind of odd metamorphosis, taking on a life of its own. I was bulging profusely by week four. My belly stuck straight out in front of my body, and my skinny bird legs barely looked strong enough to support the two of us.

As I grew closer to my due date, my belly grew and grew and grew some more. To say I was "stretched" was a gross understatement. And so the changes began.

"NO! NO! NO! This is NOT happening to me. I WILL NOT allow stretch marks to make a home on my body. My belly was destined to be exposed to the sun in a cute little swimsuit!" Ahhh... the sound of naivety echoed through my veins. My pride was being tested, and my ego was growing loudly.

I ran to the store and bought every kind of cocoa butter and serum claiming to banish stretch marks. And for the next few months of pregnancy, I slathered... or should I say, caked that stuff on every day and night. I was determined to come away from that pregnancy as tight and cute as I went in.

Ok, this is me, laughing as I write this, thinking about how self-absorbed we are growing up and how the silliest things seem so important. All the while, I made it a priority to keep exercising. It didn't take long before my runs and karate matches turned into walks and diaper changes.

My daily basketball practices became shuffled aside due to fatigue and a need for naps. My healthy eating was replaced with drive-thru quickies and anything that could be consumed with one hand while holding a baby.

In addition to motherhood, we had started a company that was consuming my extra minutes. I took my son with me everywhere and began to envy his little naps in the carrier.

As the years passed, time seemed to get shorter and shorter with all my new responsibilities. I was cooking, cleaning, changing diapers, working, building a business, and doing my best to be a great mom, wife, and boss lady. But I have to admit, in all of my effort to be the perfect woman.... I was EXHAUSTED! And trying to keep up with the social media presence of perfection I had created was a full-time job.

It wasn't long before all the responsibilities became seemingly more important than my fitness. I began noticing that my exercise habits slipped, and I worked out only when I had the time. I made it my priority to have my "to-do" list completed each day, which included everyone's needs but my own.

Suddenly, I could relate to those ladies I swore I would never become.

In a grand attempt to regain my mental and physical strength, I joined a men's basketball league. I was once an all-star basketball player and vowed that I would play till I was old and grey.

The first day I stepped back onto the court, I still had my three-point shot, and I could hustle the court like usual. Things seemed to be going great till I realized that my Kegel exercises should have been more important to me during pregnancy! The guys on the court would look at me and say, "What's up with you running to the bathroom all the time?" I wanted to slap those boys silly (in love, of course) and say, "Excuse me. When was the last time you gave birth to a watermelon?"

After my third trip to the bathroom during that first game, I looked in the mirror and shouted, "Hello! Who are you, and what have you done with my body?" It was at that moment that I knew I had a choice to make. I could either submit to the process of time and let my body take me where it chooses, or I could take massive action to show my body who was in charge. I knew, at that second, that one day I would either look back in regret and say, "I wish I had stayed in shape. " Or I would confidently say, "I'm sure glad I did!"

Of course, I would like to tell you that I stuck to my "get fit" plan, but in light of my integrity and desire to fulfill "Thou Shalt Not Lie", I must tell you the truth. I struggled. I wanted to eat like a teenager and look like a teenager. But the reality was that I wasn't that little girl anymore.

My metabolism had changed. I had new hormonal patterns, and my body was requiring something different, and I knew it. The big shift in my body, my energy, and career was happening. The fast food that used to fall off my body suddenly decided to stick to me and hold on for dear life.

Before having babies, I could get lean in a week, ready for summer fun! Now, it seemed like I needed a few months just to get in gear. I would try various exercise regimens only to feel the weight linger.

That's when I adopted a new motto:

"If you can't lose it... decorate it!"

I went to the store of "bling" and bought all kinds of sparkly belts, shirts, and other accessories to mask my extra jelly rolls of skin. To the outside world, no one would ever know of my hidden secrets, but to me, the extra weight was etching away at my confidence, my sex appeal, and even my joy. And thus began the journey of metamorphosis.

I had a choice. Succumb to the enemy, of "average," and be a byproduct of age, stress, and hormonal changes, or take dominion over my life and begin to steward my time, body, health, and wellness in a way that pleases God and serves as a living example of what it means to age gracefully... the Kingdom way.

Fast forward two decades. I am now in my fifties. My body has changed. My face has aged. But something unexpected happened along the way.

I am healthier than I have ever been. My energy is stronger. My confidence is deeper. And my understanding of how the body works has been completely transformed.

This book was born out of that journey.

Am I in the BEST shape of my life? YOU BETTER BELIEVE IT! And not because of the size of the jeans I wear. Our family is blessed because together, we live, not according to the patterns of this world, but we live in a state of total abundance... spirit, soul, and body.

I am no longer striving for perfection, but am being perfected daily by a loving God who knows exactly what we need at every stage of life. The title of this book, "FUELED," is not just about the fuel we consume, but the source of what fuels our direction, wisdom, peace, and approval.

WHAT FUELS YOU?

For years, I was Fueled by performance, perfection, a pristine figure, and the approval of others. Today, life is different. I pursue peace above all else. And after all of the years of thinking the mirror was my truth, I now see the mirror of God's word to be my constant. He makes all things beautiful in His time. This book is merely a tool to kick-start your journey to a better, healthier you.

This book is not a medical manual. It is a guide. A tool designed to help you begin a journey back to the life your body, mind, and spirit were created to live.

While I am not a physician, the principles in this book have been carefully reviewed and supported by Irina Chifor, DipION BANT CNHC, a certified nutritionist and nutritional therapist trained extensively in the principles of functional medicine. Irina's clinical practice has helped clients around the world restore their health through evidence-based nutritional therapy and functional wellness practices.

Together, grounded in the wisdom of Scripture and supported by sound nutritional science, we have assembled the principles you will discover throughout these pages. Our hope is simple. That this book awakens you. That it challenges you.

And that it helps you become a faithful steward of the temple God entrusted to you by strengthening the seven pillars of wellness that support a flourishing life.

THE DIVINE RESET

You don't need another diet. You need a divine reset.

For years, I watched people spend thousands of dollars chasing health. Diets. Powders. Pills. Programs. Yet the results were always the same. Weight returned. Energy crashed. Frustration grew. Why? Because most health systems focus on treating symptoms rather than restoring design.

This book is not about another diet. It is about realignment.

Because 95% of diets fail. Not because people are lazy or lack willpower, but because they're missing the true source of lasting change. This book is not about restriction. It's about realignment. You were never designed to operate on willpower alone. You were created to live Fueled by the Spirit of God, and that is where transformation begins.

When the Holy Spirit becomes the life coach of your consciousness, every decision you make is filtered through Kingdom wisdom. Your appetite shifts. Your cravings lose power. Your thoughts align with Truth. And your body, yes, even your cells and hormones, begin to align with divine order.

This is Heaven's blueprint for total wellness. It's the reason people who have followed this framework have lost hundreds of pounds, reversed chronic symptoms, healed emotionally, and come alive spiritually. In this book, you'll be introduced to the 7 Pillars of Optimal Wellness:

1. **Spiritual Fitness** – You are a spirit first, living inside a human body.
2. **Mental Mastery** – Learn to renew your mind and take every thought captive.
3. **Hydration** – Water is life. Your cells are thirsty for more than you realize.
4. **Nutrition** – Fuel that honors the temple God gave you.
5. **Rest** – Healing happens when the body is allowed to recover.
6. **Movement** – Your body was designed to move.
7. **The Jesus Way** – A life of wholeness that flows from intimacy with Christ.

Together, these pillars create a comprehensive framework that honors how God designed you... spirit, soul, and body to function as one integrated system. You'll also learn how your hormones, mitochondria, and cellular health play key roles in how you feel, and how to stop fighting your body and start partnering with it.

SETTING FUELED GOALS

A dream without a plan is simply wishful thinking.

As you read this book and begin applying the principles of the Fueled lifestyle, it is important to define what success looks like for you. Clear goals create clarity of action. When you know where you are going, your daily choices begin to align with that direction.

SET CLEAR, ACTIONABLE GOALS FOR THE PROGRAM

Example: "I want to lose 50 lbs. in the next five months." (That is 10 pounds per month or approximately 2-3 pounds per week on average.) By having measurable goals and a specific timeframe, you can reverse engineer your goals into bite-sized milestones that give you weekly celebrations.

What are your top three goals for the Fueled program?

Goal 1: ____________________________________
What actionable steps will you need to take?

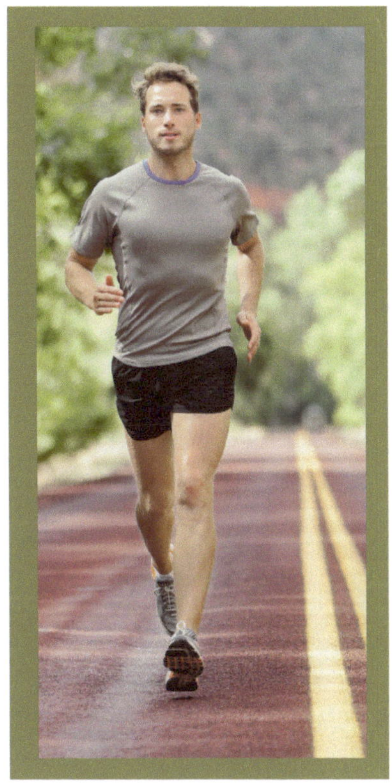

Goal 2: ____________________________________
What actionable steps will you need to take?

Goal 3: ____________________________________
What actionable steps will you need to take?

Before we begin, say this out loud:

I will never be the same again. Holy Spirit, have Your way with me. Mold me into the temple Your Spirit was born to inhabit. I say yes to Your will, and I choose to walk in Your ways. In Jesus' name, Amen.

YOUR SEVEN-DAY FUELED AUDIT

For the next seven days, simply observe your current habits, including foods, drinks, water, gum, candy, medicines, etc. Consider the hours you spend on social media, TV, empty conversations, etc. Fill out this audit to raise awareness of what you need to work on. You may need to use a separate notebook to take more details.

	Sunday	Monday	Tuesday	Wednesday	Thursday	Friday	Saturday
What did you eat?							
How much water did you drink?							
How often did you look at social media?							
How often did you pray or meditate?							
What did you do for physical exercise?							
On a scale of 1-10 how stressful was your day?							
How often did you stop and express gratitude?							
On a scale of 1-10, what was your energy level?							
How much sleep did you get each night?							
How often did you say grace before eating?							

Did you eat anything after 6 p.m. this week? If so, what was it and at what time?______________________________

____

COMMITMENT TO EXCELLENCE

I, ______________________________, commit to completing this journey of transformation. I invite the Holy Spirit to guide, challenge, and strengthen me daily.

I recognize that lasting change requires action. By choosing to steward my body, my time, and my health according to God's design, I position myself and my family for a life of strength, vitality, and purpose. I will not settle for average. I will pursue excellence in how I care for the temple God has entrusted to me.

I recognize that the enemy of my destiny does not want me to finish strong. He has been at this game of sabotaging God's people for thousands of years, and I am not so foolish as to think I can take him on alone. That is why I choose to gain wisdom in counsel and align myself with the coaches of this program and the accountability partner I choose to be my confidant in this journey. I will not only start this plan for optimal wellness, but I will finish strong and become the leader of health, wealth, and vitality I was destined to be.

Today's Date: _________________________ Current Weight: _________________________

PERSONAL AFFIRMATION

Write a statement of your ideal future.

____

____

____

____

Signature: ____ Date: ____________________

Accountability Partner: ____

An olive tree does not flourish overnight.

It flourishes because its roots grow deeper season after season.

PART TWO:
ROOTED

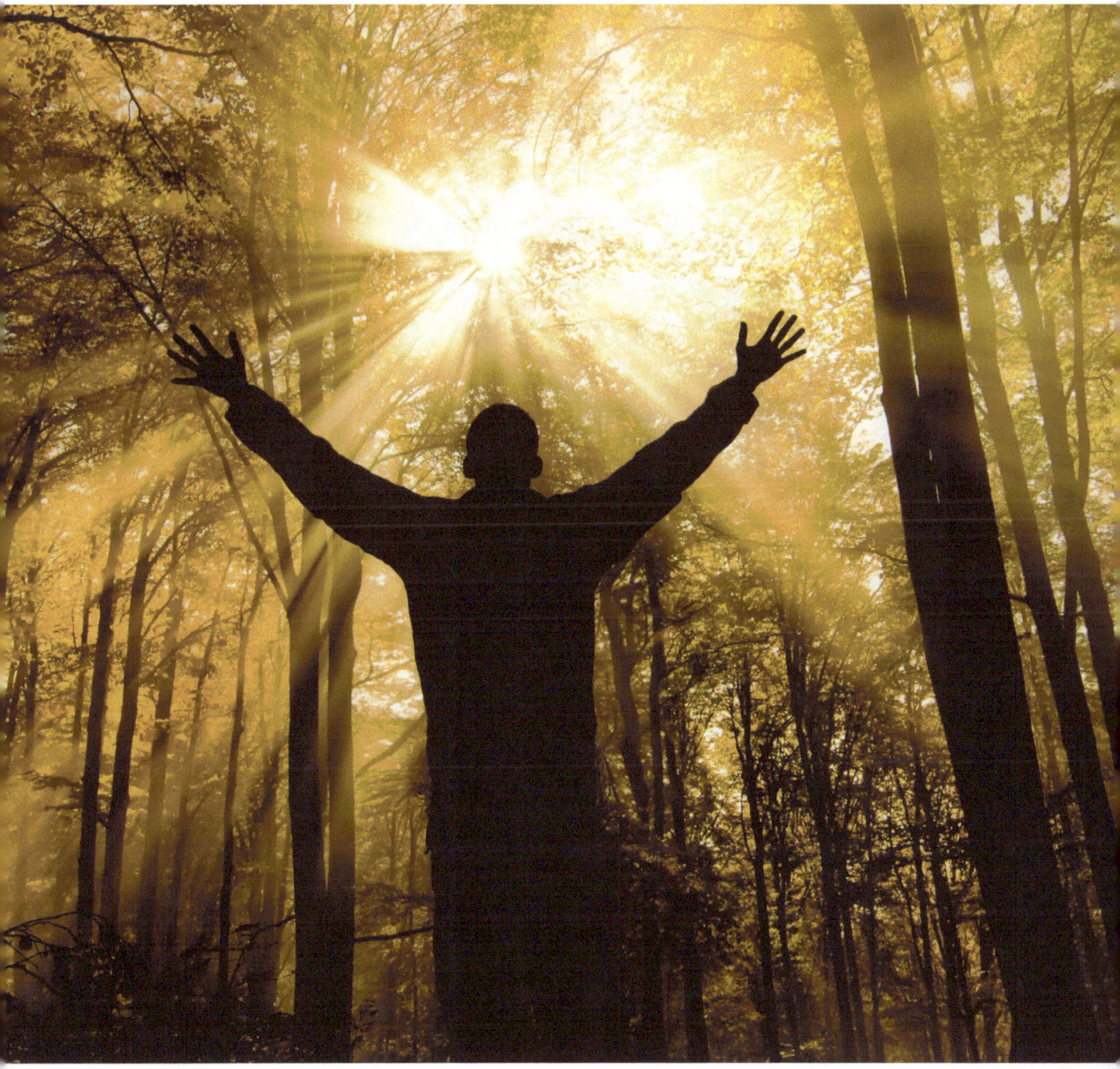

"Do not conform to the pattern of this world,
but be transformed by the renewing of your mind."
— **Romans 12:2**

PILLAR 1: SPIRITUAL FITNESS

NEW LIFE BEGINS FROM WITHIN

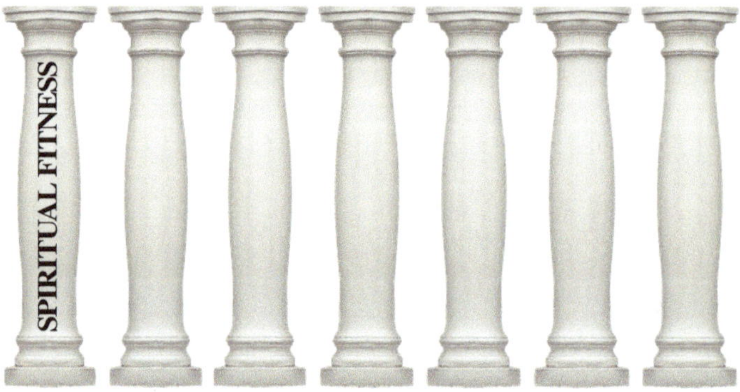

"This means that anyone who belongs to Christ has become a new person. The old life is gone; a new life has begun!"
— 2 Corinthians 5:17

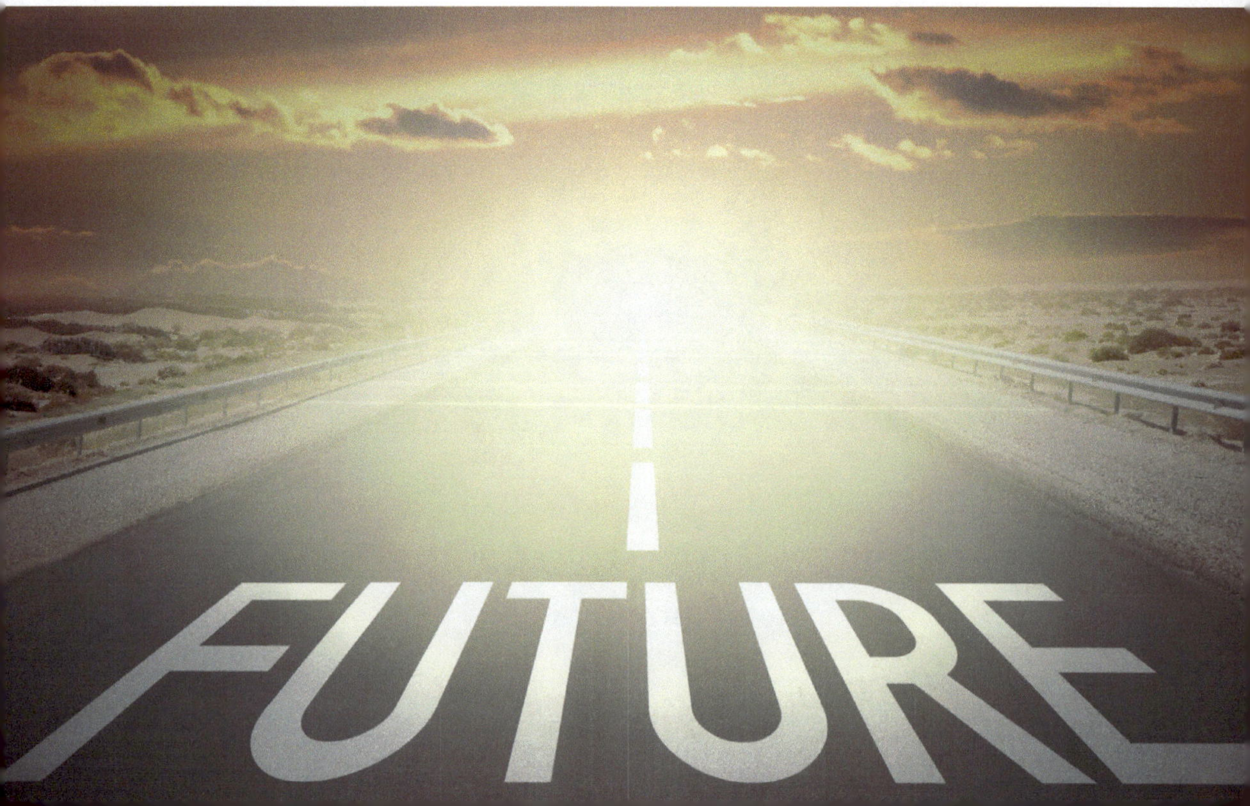

CHAPTER 1

BELIEVING THE TRUTH

"In the beginning, God created."

Let that land. Those first five words in Genesis hold more wisdom than any wellness trend on Instagram.

Right there is your first clue.

Who created the body? God.
Who holds the blueprint for optimal health? God.
Who should we look to for healing, energy, and wholeness? God.

Not TikTok.
Not the latest juice cleanse.
God.

What if Scripture held the real blueprint for success?

Not just spiritually.
But physically.
Emotionally.
Even financially.

Let's start exactly where God did... in the beginning.

Unfortunately, most wellness programs start in the middle of the story. They obsess over macros, muscle mass, or biohacks (which, let's be honest, sound more like something out of a sci-fi film than a wellness plan). And while those things have value, they miss the foundation.

You are a spirit being having a temporary human experience inside a beautifully flawed and divinely designed body. Any plan that skips over the spirit is already off course. Yes, your biochemistry matters. Yes, your body is an incredible instrument of praise.

But true transformation starts in the spirit, not in your supplement cabinet. That's why God, in His infinite brilliance, gave us more than a survival guide. He gave us the Bible, a divine constitution. A Kingdom blueprint. A full-access guide to living in wholeness and authority right here on Earth.

Some people call it the Basic Instructions Before Leaving Earth.

I call it the ultimate wellness manual and the constitution of the Kingdom of God. It is a constitution given to us straight from the Manufacturer. And throughout this journey, we're going to do what Jesus did, and that is to apply Kingdom principles to everyday life. We're going to reclaim dominion over our bodies, our appetites, our time, our energy, and yes, our health. Because God didn't design you to barely survive. He created you to thrive. And if we're going to begin at the beginning, we must begin where all real transformation begins... with faith.

NOW FAITH

Faith Has Weight.

Let's set something straight... Faith isn't wishful thinking. It isn't crossing your fingers and hoping something works out someday.

Faith is substance.

It is real.
It carries weight.
And it exists now.

Hebrews 11:1 tells us: "Now faith is the substance of things hoped for, the evidence of things not seen."

Did you catch that?

NOW faith.

Not someday, faith. Not "once I lose the weight" faith.

Faith lives in the present. It carries the evidence of what has not yet manifested. That means when you walk by faith, you are not hoping for transformation.

You are standing in it. Speaking from it. Living like it is already done. Because in the Kingdom, it is.

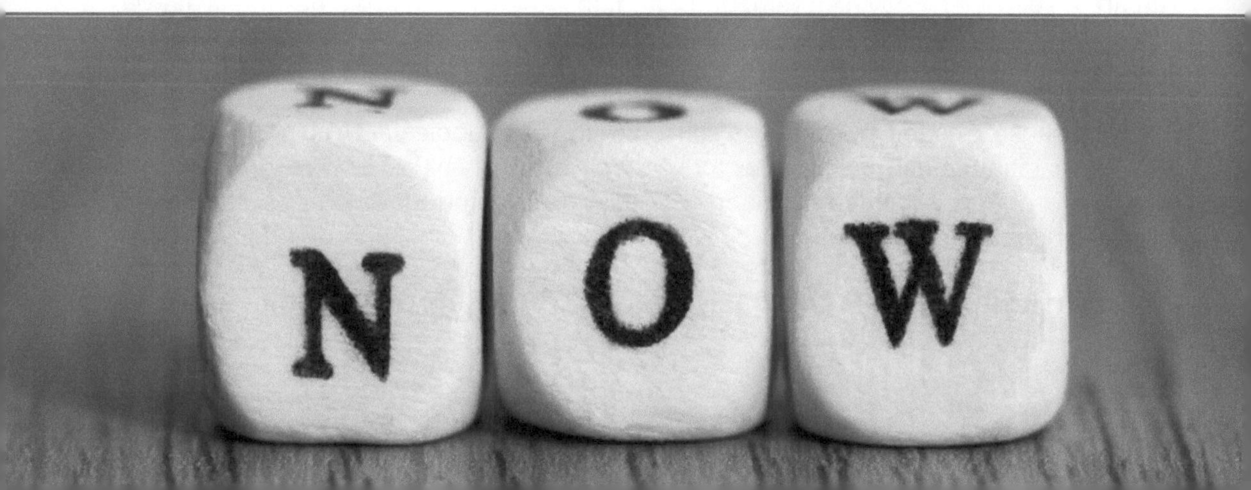

Activate Your Faith

How much do you weigh?

No, not today. Not what the scale says right now. What is the weight you believe for? The weight you see by faith. Write it down. Claim it. Declare it. Own it.

My Faith Weight: ________________

Now ask yourself a deeper question.

Who is the person who lives at that weight?
What kind of energy do they carry?
What kind of discipline do they practice?
What kind of confidence do they walk in?

Write Your Faith Identity

At my faith weight I am someone who: ______________________________

____

____

____

Close your eyes. See yourself carrying that weight with confidence, energy, and strength. Feel it. Thank God for it. Walk in it.

Because faith does not wait for results to believe.

Faith believes... and then the results show up.

Now imagine your life from that place.

How is your life different now that you are at your faith weight?
How does it impact your family?
What are you able to do differently?
How does it affect your ability to steward the ideas, creativity, and gifts God has placed in you?

It is from that vision that we begin to rebuild your wholeness, spirit, soul, and body.

HUMAN CONSCIOUSNESS
VS.
SUPER CONSCIOUSNESS

"Set your mind on things above, not on earthly things."
— Colossians 3:2

The Problem With Human Consciousness

In all my years of coaching and consulting, I've come to one unshakable truth: true wellness, real life transformation, starts in the spirit. Not in the gym. Not on the plate. Not even in the mind. The body follows the spirit.

When your spirit is aligned with God, your mind comes into order, your hormones stabilize, your cravings shift, and your life begins to reflect Kingdom peace. That's why Spiritual Fitness is not just the first pillar—it's the cornerstone.

And the Holy Spirit made this abundantly clear to me one night in a dream.

The Dream: The 40th Floor and Above

In the dream, I stood on the first floor of a towering building. The lights were off. Darkness surrounded me. The atmosphere was heavy, silent, and thick with despair.

I looked around and saw people curled up on the ground in the fetal position. They were not lazy. They were not weak. They were emotionally numb and weighed down by fear, anxiety, grief, and hopelessness.

They were exhausted. Spiritually crushed.

I stepped into an elevator. As the elevator rose, the atmosphere on each floor changed. Each level revealed a different way people search for meaning, healing, and success.

The next floor glowed red.

It was filled with high-powered individuals, CEOs, influencers, athletes, and executives. This floor pulsed with ambition and ego.

The people were driven, but the drive came from a dark place: greed, power, performance, and addiction to success. It looked successful, but it felt empty. The leaders there were searching for success but starving for greater significance. They were toiling and striving in beast mode but missing the mark of God's best mode for their lives.

There were doctors, lawyers, pastors, coaches, teachers, athletes, and masses of people driven by a spirit of performance and competition.

The next floor was cast in a blue hue.

This was the floor of rules, political divisions, religious dogma, and tribal thinking. It was orderly but rigid. Judgment and superiority filled the air. People were segmented by belief systems, each claiming to be right. Love was conditional. Truth was limited by dogma.

On the next floor, the light shifted to green.

These were "earth energy" people. They were kind, thoughtful, peaceful. They honored nature, protected animals, and advocated for justice. But their hope was rooted in creation, not the Creator. It was beautiful, but misdirected. They honored creation but had lost connection with the Creator.

The next floor seemed to be the highest of them all and was drenched in orange light.

It was dazzling. Wealthy. Powerful. It looked like the pinnacle of human success. It seemed to have everything money could buy. There was even an element of earthly love and collaboration. Think Oprah. Elon. Global leaders with money, fame, and influence.

This was the 39th floor. The highest level human effort could reach. The world would call it the pinnacle of success. But God had something else to show me.

As the elevator rose, I began to see a pattern. Each floor was Fueled by something different.

THE ELEVATOR OF
SPIRITUAL TRANSCENDENCE

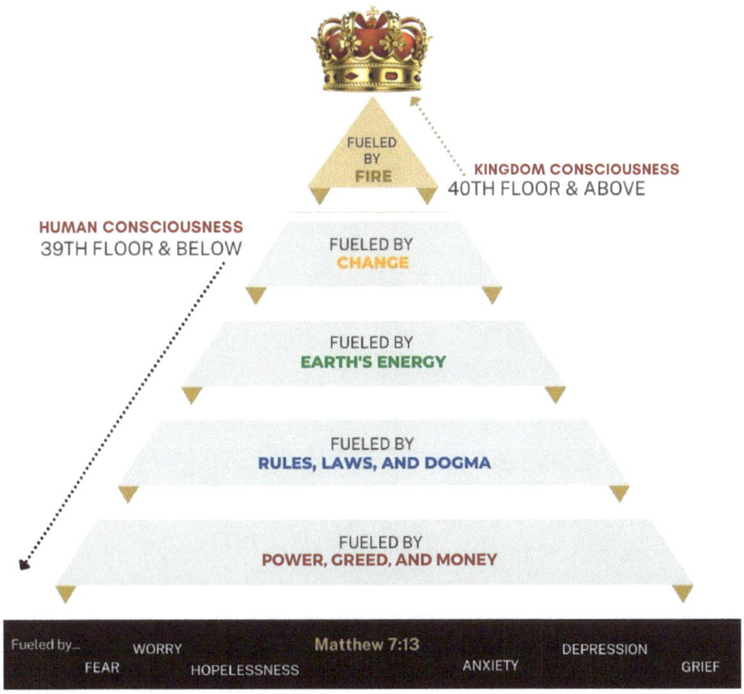

As I stood there on the 39th floor, admiring the glow of it all, I heard the voice of God say:

"Step out of the elevator and look to your right."

I obeyed.

And there it was, another elevator that seemed to be "next-level," like a penthouse elevator. It was smaller. More elegant. Radiant with a different kind of light. Above it, a sign read: **"The 40th Floor and Above."**

I walked toward it and noticed it didn't have buttons, only a slot for a card reader.

I looked down and saw a card in my hand.

Etched into the metal was one name:

JESUS

As I slid the card in, the door opened.

Light poured out. It was not just natural light, but something deeper. It illuminated everything. I stepped in, and the elevator lifted me to a place words can hardly describe.

THE 40TH FLOOR
KINGDOM CONSCIOUSNESS

When the doors opened, I had arrived at the Kingdom floor of Heaven on Earth.

This was the realm of divine consciousness. The presence of God filled the atmosphere. Everything moved in harmony with His nature.

Love.
Joy.
Peace.
Patience.
Kindness.
Goodness.
Faithfulness.
Gentleness.
Self-control.

This was the mind of Christ.

The Fruit of the Spirit wasn't just present here. It was the very atmosphere. This was the mind of Christ. This was divine health, wholeness, and clarity. This was what it meant to live spirit-first.

And again, I heard the Father say: *"Keep your mind on things above, not on earthly things."*

Why the 40th Floor Matters

Most wellness programs begin on the 39th floor and try to work their way downward.

They focus on treating symptoms such as weight gain, brain fog, low energy, and hormone imbalance while overlooking the root issue.

But real transformation requires going deeper than the symptoms. We must ask why they exist in the first place. And more often than people realize, the cause is not merely physical. It is connected to a spiritual gap that has never been addressed.

When the human spirit is disconnected from the Spirit of God, everything begins to drift out of alignment. Thoughts become cluttered. Emotions spiral. The body carries the burden. Decisions begin to flow from fear instead of faith.

True wellness does not begin with religious performance or trying harder. It begins with divine alignment.

It is the process of training your spirit to hear God, respond in obedience, and walk in the authority He designed you to carry.

Spiritual Fitness Changes Everything

When the spirit comes into alignment with God, the body begins to follow.

Hormones begin to regulate as stress gives way to peace. Mitochondria, the tiny engines that produce energy in your cells, become more efficient when the body rests in God's design. Cellular health improves as the nervous system settles in the presence of God.

This is what happens when spiritual fitness becomes the foundation. Your life begins to overflow with Kingdom wellness, where spirit, soul, and body move back into the harmony they were created to experience.

So if you have been living on the lower floors, do not lose heart. Whether the fuel in your life has been fear, guilt, greed, performance, judgment, or even worldly success, there is still an invitation to step off that elevator.

There is a better way. There is another elevator that leads to Heaven on Earth.

And the access card?

You already have it. **His name is Jesus.**

He is the door to the 40th floor and above. The place where transformation begins and where true wellness is no longer something you chase but something you begin to live.

Because when your spirit is Fueled, your whole life begins to flourish.

HEALING THROUGH IDENTITY
METAMORPHOSIS

"Therefore, if anyone is in Christ, the new creation has come:
The old has gone, the new is here!"
— 2 Corinthians 5:17

There is a heaviness you cannot quite explain.

You cleaned up your eating. You committed to the gym. You bought the vitamins and downloaded the apps. And yet something still feels heavy.

Not in your body. In your soul.

A spiritual kind of weight that does not respond to willpower, workouts, or green juice.

This is the weight of an unhealed identity.

The echo of trauma, betrayal, fear, or disappointment that was never fully processed, only buried.

If this resonates, you are not alone. This is exactly where many people get stuck on their wellness journey. But this is also where God begins His deepest work of transformation.

JUST BREATHE

Before we begin the work ahead, I invite you to be still.

Put on soft Christian meditation music or instrumental worship that is peaceful and free of lyrics. Sit somewhere quiet and comfortable.

Close your eyes.

Focus on your breath.

Inhale slowly. Exhale deeply.

Let your breath move like the rhythm of ocean waves.

Steady.
Constant.
Healing.

Breathing itself is an exchange. Carbon dioxide leaves. Oxygen enters. Darkness gives way to light.

With each inhale, imagine breathing in everything that flows from the 40th floor and above. With each exhale, release the weight of the 39th floor and below.

INHALE
Breathe in love, joy, peace, and the fruit of the Spirit.

EXHALE
Release pressure, shame, fear, and the lies you have carried.

INHALE
Patience, kindness, and faithfulness.

EXHALE
Limiting beliefs, toxic expectations, and the weight of past failures.

Take ten deep, intentional breaths.

With each breath, feel yourself releasing false labels and stepping into sacred stillness.

"Come to me, all who are weary and burdened, and I will give you rest."
— Matthew 11:28

Now we begin.

FROM REVELATION TO RESTORATION

Now that we understand the difference between human consciousness and Kingdom consciousness, the question becomes personal.

How do we actually step into the life God designed?

Transformation rarely begins with behavior. It begins with identity. Many people try to change their habits without ever healing the wounds the labels they carry inflict. But if identity remains wounded, behavior eventually returns to the same patterns.

God does not begin with performance. He begins with identity.

Before we strengthen the pillars of wellness, we must release the false names we have carried and rediscover the identity God has spoken over our lives.

This is where healing begins.

SPIRITUAL IDENTITY AUDIT

STEP ONE: ASSESS

Open your journal or use the timeline chart provided.

You are about to walk back through your life. Not to relive the pain, but to release the weight that has been shaping your identity.

Many of us unknowingly build our identity around moments that wounded us.

A harsh word.
A betrayal.
A loss.
A divorce.
A childhood trauma.
A label spoken over us in anger or fear.
Or even addiction.

These moments become identity markers. They shape how we see ourselves, even when God never intended that label for our lives.

Maybe someone spoke words of shame, rejection, or poverty over you.

Maybe a painful event carved a message into your soul that whispered, "You are not enough."

Using the timeline on the next page, begin writing down the significant moments that shaped your identity, both positive and painful.

These are the mile markers of your story.

We've worked with countless men and women who were molested as children and carried that trauma like an invisible cloak. It followed them into every relationship, decision, and mirror they looked into. They saw themselves as broken instead of healed.

Too often, we wear an identity shaped by history rather than the identity we've been given through Christ. But that changes today. We are not victims of our past. We are vessels of His purpose. Let's uncover those old identity markers and step into the life God has prepared for us.

Look at the timeline on the next page. Take as long as you need.

Allow the Holy Spirit to guide this process.

Breathe. Pause. Write.

MY TIMELINE

Birth

Negative Memories

Positive Memories

Today

STEP TWO: ADDRESS

How does God see these mile markers in your life?

Once your timeline is complete, review each event and ask for God's perspective and how He can use them for His glory.

I once led this exercise with 14 high-achieving women from one of the largest insurance companies in the U.S. Each of them was a multi-million-dollar producer. From the outside, they were the definition of "having it all." But within 15 minutes of writing the timeline, the room was filled with tears.

One woman broke the silence with a story that stunned the room.

She had been driving her daughter to the museum when a truck hydroplaned and struck them head-on. Her toddler was thrown from the car and died in her arms on the side of the road. The room fell silent.

And yet I knew God was not finished with her story.

I gently asked, "Would you be willing to let God use that moment?"
Through tears, she whispered yes.

I asked her to imagine the day again, not to relive it, but to redeem it. Then I asked her to hold her baby girl one more time and make a promise.

She whispered, "I will be your voice. I will live with passion and purpose so that your name lives on."

That day, she reidentified.

She was no longer the mother defined by loss.
She became a voice of hope for grieving families.
Her deepest pain became a Kingdom assignment.

This is the power of addressing your identity markers through the eyes of the Holy Spirit.

STEP THREE: APPLY GOD'S WORD

God never wastes a wound. Romans 8:28 tells us that He works ALL THINGS together for good to them that love God and are called according to His purpose. That means that no matter what you've gone through, God can use it to be a stepping stone in your destiny and use it to bring hope, help, and healing to others. Your job isn't to fix the past. It's to give it to God and let Him reframe it in light of eternity.

Once you've gone through each marker and asked how God can use it for His good, you're ready to begin shifting your mind from old things to new beginnings. This is essential in living a life of total wellness rooted in a Kingdom identity.

Look at your timeline. List any significant life lessons that you have learned about yourself, God, and others. How can that milestone create value that brings healing to others in the future?

Memory	Lesson	Value

Review your timeline again. Are there areas of unforgiveness that have become roots of bitterness, fear, depression, or anxiety?

Take a moment now to release those anchors to God. Forgive those who have hurt you This is the Kingdom way.

Pray this prayer: *Father God, I give these areas of pain and weakness to You. Forgive me for anything I have done that allowed them to separate me from Your will and Your best for my life.*

I am not defined by my past. I choose to identify with You and the new beginning You offer. Amen.

Your past may explain your story, but it does not define your identity. In Christ, the story is still being written.

PILLAR 2:
MENTAL MASTERY

TAKING EVERY THOUGHT CAPTIVE

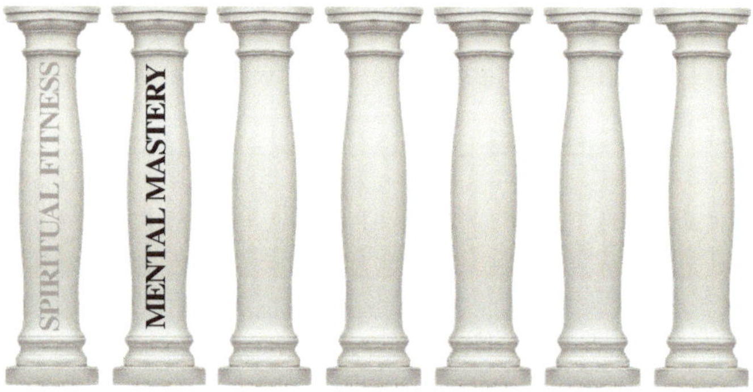

"I focus on this one thing:
Forgetting the past and looking forward to what lies ahead."
— Philippians 3:13

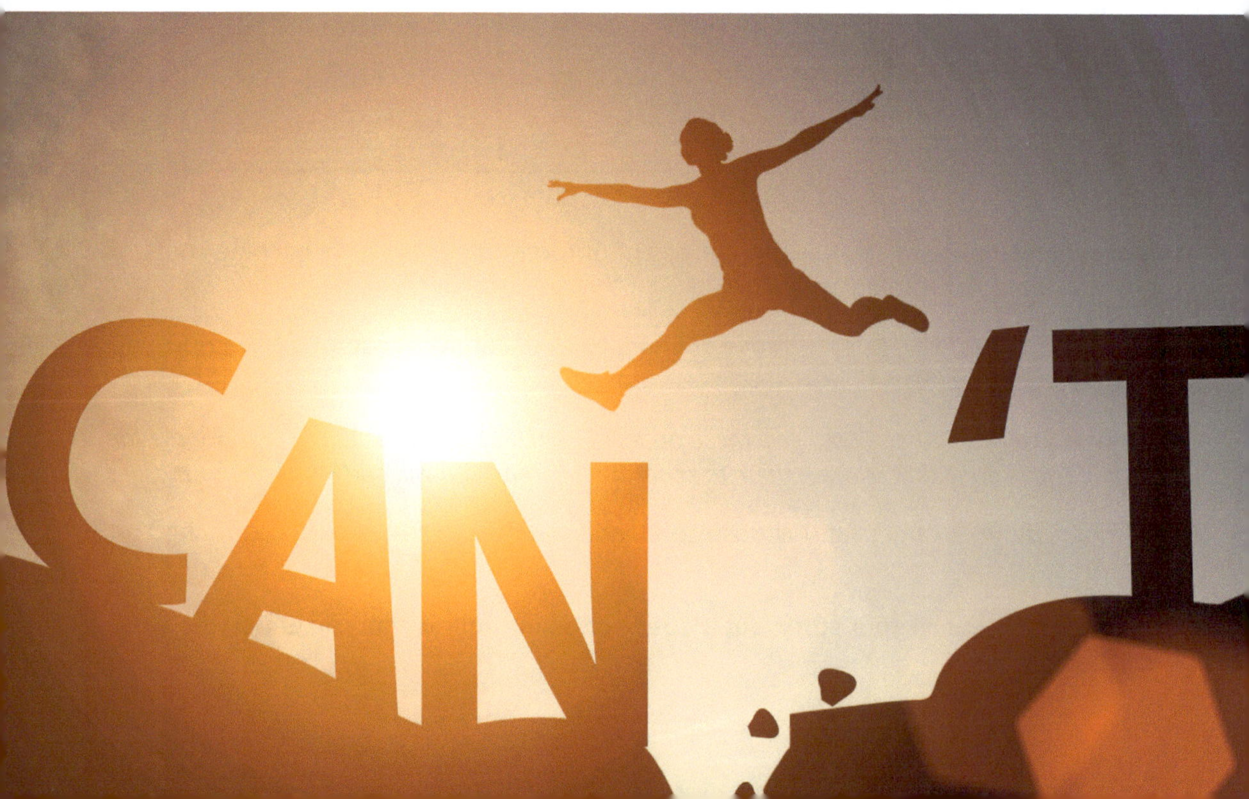

CHAPTER 2

EMOTIONAL HIJACKING

Today is the day you stop tiptoeing around transformation and finally make a decisive shift. This is your invitation to step into dominion and authority. Not only over your weight, your workouts, or your water intake, but over your past, your present, and your future.

Your identity in Christ is more than a spiritual status upgrade. It is your weapon against the old voices of the enemy.

As you practice living from the 40th floor and above, you will begin to see clearly. This is the place of divine alignment, Kingdom perspective, and the mind of Christ. And soon you will realize something important.

The real battlefield is not in your body. It is in your mind.

And the enemy has been targeting that battlefield for thousands of years.

In my book *UNLEASHED* and Anointed for Kingdom Business, I talk about lice and insects and how they were one of the greatest threats to sheep in Biblical times.

It was not lions or bears that killed the most sheep. It was the tiny parasites that crawled into their ears and infested their brains, slowly destroying them from the inside out.

The same thing happens in the human mind. If the enemy cannot steal your salvation, he will try to hijack your thinking. That is why spiritual warfare rarely looks dramatic. It looks like mental exhaustion. It sounds like whispers in the background of your thoughts.

"You will never change."
"This is just who you are."
"Why even try?"

Sound familiar?

Our culture has responded to this crisis with labels, diagnoses, and prescriptions for anxiety, depression, ADHD, and bipolar disorder. Medication has its place, but we must also recognize something deeper.

Many people are fighting a spiritual battle with purely physical tools.

A recent Deloitte study revealed that mental health costs already exceed 477 billion dollars each year and are projected to reach 1.3 trillion by 2040.

This is not just a healthcare issue. It is a spiritual crisis.

LET TRANSFORMATION BEGIN...

"Be transformed by the renewing of your mind."
— Romans 12:2

Transformation does not happen through sheer effort. It does not come through toxic positivity or motivational slogans.

True and lasting change happens when the mind is renewed, aligned, and rewired to match Heaven's truth.

When we surrender fear, pride, worry, and doubt, we stop living like rag dolls tossed in a whirlwind of emotion.

You were not created for emotional roller coasters. You were created to think like Christ.

To rule your thoughts with the Word of God.
To discern His voice from the noise of the world.
To reject lies and replace them with truth.

That is how dominion begins.

Your thoughts shape your wellness.

Your words shape your outcomes.

Mental health will always influence physical health because thoughts become patterns, and patterns become lives.

Here is the hard truth.

You can eat clean, drink your water, and work out six days a week. But if your mind is still rehearsing shame, fear, and failure, you are strengthening the body while starving the soul.

Mindset is not fluff.
It is foundational.

A mind rooted in Kingdom truth is one of the most powerful tools in your wellness journey.

How you see yourself, your circumstances, and your future will either fuel your healing or quietly sabotage it.

Taking dominion over your thoughts is not simply a matter of shifting your mindset.
It is renewing your mind.
And you don't have to do it alone.

You have the mind of Christ.

Make this declaration today:

I no longer conform to the patterns of this world. I am transformed by the renewing of my mind. I take every thought captive and make it obedient to Christ. Fear no longer leads me. Faith leads me. I have the mind of Christ. I steward my thoughts with power, love, and a sound mind.

TAKE DOMINION OVER YOUR MIND

Think of your mind like a running playlist. You can choose what is streaming at any given time. Thousands of songs are available, but only a few should make it into your personal playlist.

The same is true of your thoughts. You can control what you play on repeat. Just because a thought appears does not mean it belongs on your playlist.

Your job is to decide which thoughts get replayed, which thoughts get deleted, and which thoughts are replaced with truth. Mental mastery begins when you realize this powerful truth: **You are the curator of your mind. You choose what you think.**

"Finally, brothers and sisters, whatever is true, whatever is noble, whatever is right, whatever is pure, whatever is lovely, whatever is admirable, if anything is excellent or praiseworthy, think about such things."
— Philippians 4:8

Throughout Scripture, we see King David doing something quite amazing that pulled him out of some very desperate times.

He talked to himself. He spoke to his own soul.

In Psalm 42:5, he writes, *"Why, my soul, are you downcast? Why so disturbed within me? Put your hope in God."*

Notice what David is doing. He is not surrendering to the emotion. He is confronting it.

His soul is discouraged. His thoughts are heavy. But instead of letting those thoughts take control, he interrupts them and redirects his mind back toward God.

David understood that the mind will often drift toward fear, grief, and discouragement if it is left unchecked.

So he did something powerful. He led his thoughts. He changed his playlist!

THE BATTLEFIELD OF THE MIND

We process over 6,000 thoughts each day. This vast number underscores why scripture emphasizes the importance of renewing our minds daily. It's essential to pause and consider what governs your actions. Often, it's not physical hunger that leads us to eat, but emotional and mental hungers linked to our thoughts and feelings.

Reflect on the voices that resonate within you. Are they aligned with your identity in Christ, or do they pull you away from it? On the form below, list the recurring thoughts in your mind that have been holding you back.

____

____

Are those voices affirming your true identity in Christ and His promises, or are they undermining your divine purpose and peace?

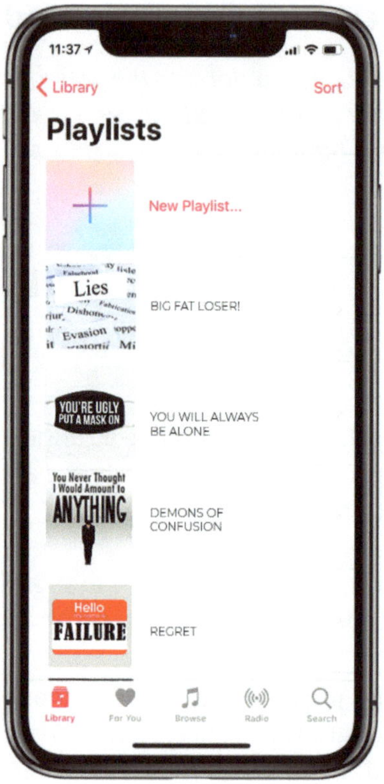

RETRAIN YOUR BRAIN

Out with the old... In with the new!

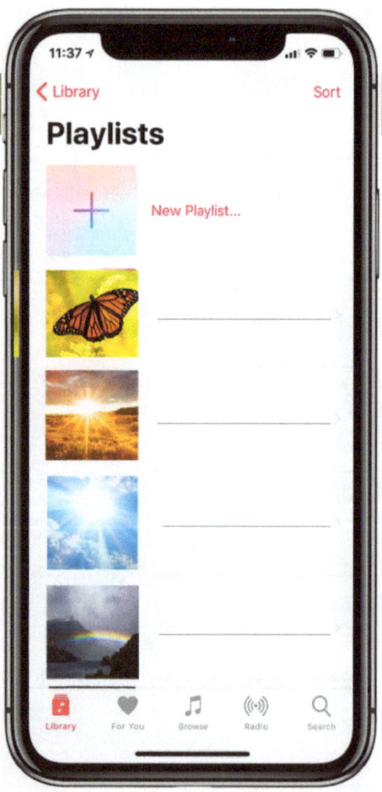

Now, take time to replace that old playlist with new affirmations for life, love, hope, and faith. What do you want to tell the spirit living inside of your body? What words do you want to set on replay?

____

____

____

____

"This means that anyone who belongs to Christ has become a new person. The old life is gone; a new life has begun!"
— 2 Corinthians 5:17

HUMAN CONDITIONING

Several years ago, the Denver Zoo received a large polar bear but had no proper habitat prepared for it. Building the new enclosure would take several years, so temporarily the bear was placed in a small holding cage measuring only twelve feet by twelve feet.

Inside that confined space the bear could take only three steps in any direction before reaching a barrier. Three years later the new habitat was finally complete. It was expansive, beautiful, and designed to give the bear freedom to roam. But something unexpected happened.

Even with all that open space, the bear continued to walk only three steps at a time.

Back and forth. Back and forth.

Although the cage was gone, the conditioning remained. The bear had internalized the limits of its old environment.

Many people live the same way.

Long after the limitations of their past are removed, they still walk within the boundaries their minds learned years ago.

This is why the Apostle Paul wrote:

"Do not conform to the pattern of this world,
but be transformed by the renewing of your mind."
— Romans 12:2

Transformation begins when the mind learns to live beyond its old cage.

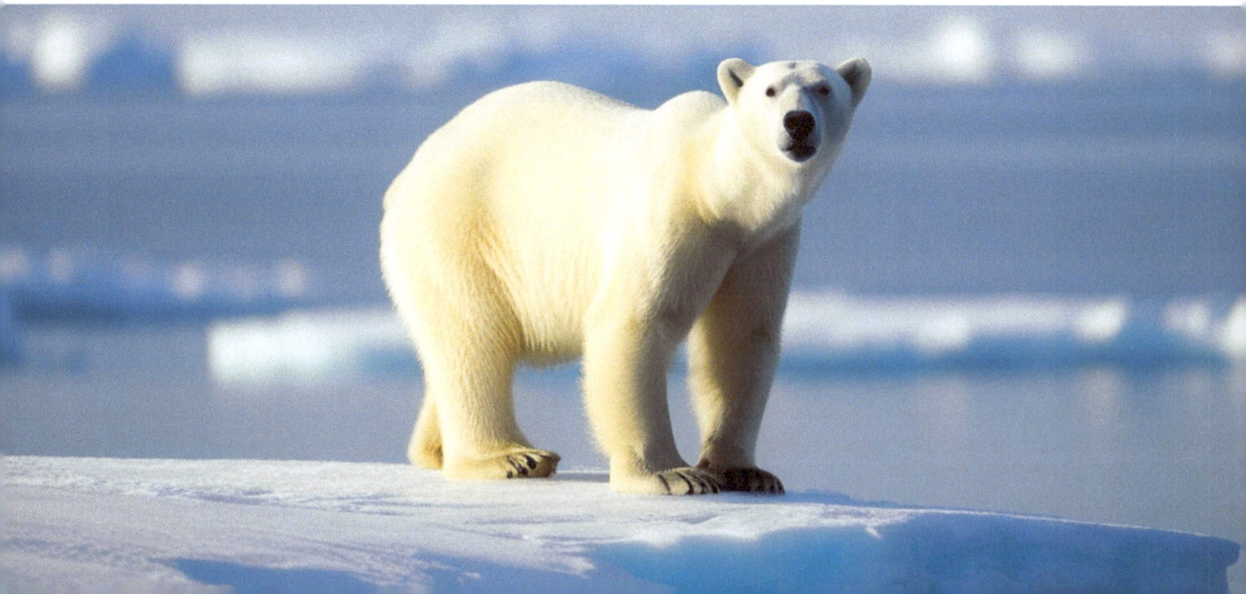

THE WONDER OF YOU

"Let us make mankind in our image, in our likeness, so that they will rule over the fish in the sea and the birds in the sky, over the livestock and all the wild animals, and over all the creatures that move along the ground."
— Genesis 1:26

God designed Earth to reflect Heaven. His authority, glory, and government were meant to be displayed through humanity. Adam and Eve were created as His first children and given dominion over every living thing.

Genesis 1:28 declares: *"Be fruitful and multiply and fill the earth and subdue it."*

Humanity was never meant to live powerless. We were created to carry God's authority into the world. But when Adam and Eve surrendered that dominion through disobedience, the consequences rippled through every generation. Sin introduced pain, sickness, shame, fear, and broken identity into the human experience.

Yet God did not abandon His design. Through Jesus Christ, that authority was restored.

Through His death, burial, and resurrection, the same Spirit that raised Christ from the dead now lives within every believer.

God expands His Kingdom on Earth through transformed lives. And that transformation requires a complete renewal of the spirit, soul, and body.

You are not simply flesh and bone. You carry the imprint of Heaven. You are a living vessel of spiritual potential, and when the Holy Spirit activates that potential, the limits of your past no longer define your future.

"For God has not given us a spirit of fear and timidity, but of power, love, and self-discipline."
— 2 Timothy 1:7

"Do you not know that you are the temple of God and that the Spirit of God dwells in you? If anyone defiles the temple of God, God will destroy him. For the temple of God is holy, which temple you are."
— 1 Corinthians 3:16-17

DISCOVERING THE REAL YOU

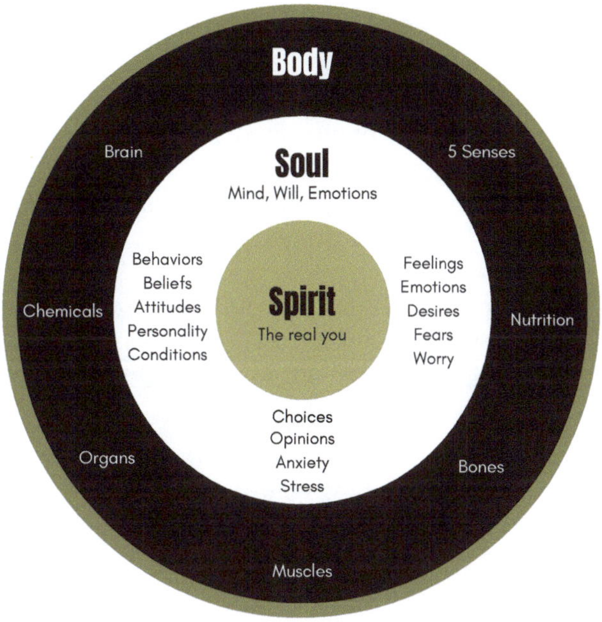

You are a spirit being living in a physical body and equipped with a mind, will, and emotions. These three together form what Scripture calls the "soul."

Your body is your earthly vessel.
Your soul is the interface through which you think, feel, and make decisions.
But your spirit is the real you.

Many people live driven primarily by emotions, fears, cravings, and temporary desires. When the body and emotions lead, decisions are shaped by impulse, comfort, or external pressure.

But when the spirit leads, life begins to align with purpose.

Your soul, like your body, is mortal. But your spirit, once reborn in Christ, carries eternal life.

Baptism symbolizes this transformation. The old life is buried, and a new life emerges.

From that moment forward, the Spirit of God within you empowers you to bring your thoughts, emotions, and physical habits into alignment with Heaven.

"Therefore, if anyone is in Christ, he is a new creation.
The old has passed away; behold, the new has come."
— 2 Corinthians 5:17

Unlike many programs that jump right into weighing your body, putting you on a treadmill, or targeting your nutrition from day one, we are going to start with THE REAL YOU, not the body of form and matter that surrounds you. By first looking at your SQ (Spiritual Quotient) and your EQ (Emotional Quotient), we can study the foundations of why you do what you do and help you identify better with the REAL YOU... the Holy Spirit-transformed you!

"Don't copy the behavior or fads of this world, but let God transform you into a new person by changing the way you think. Then you will learn to know God's will for you, which is good and pleasing and perfect."
— Romans 12:2

The goal of this program is to help you step into divine health that represents your new heaven-on-earth identity. For this to happen, you must learn to silence the voices of self-doubt, fear, unforgiveness, limiting beliefs, anxiety, and other emotions that have ruled or dominated your soul (mind, will, and emotions).

Most wellness programs begin by weighing your body.
But we are beginning somewhere deeper.

We begin with the REAL YOU.

Question 1: How much do you weigh? ________

If you wrote the number on the scale, that is simply the measurement of your body today.

Question 2: How much does the REAL YOU weigh? ________

Beneath your body mass is a spirit that is not defined by the patterns of your past.

From this moment forward, we will begin speaking to that REAL YOU.

The you who is healthy.
The you who is disciplined.
The you who carries the authority of God within.

Your body is simply the external documentation of your journey. As the REAL YOU takes leadership over your choices, your body will follow.

From this day forward, I will only speak to the REAL YOU. Yes, we will weigh and measure, but these are only external documentation of your body mass, so we can see how you are doing on your journey. As you transform and allow the REAL YOU to take dominion in your choices, your body will naturally follow.

Until now, you have probably been so "body" conscious that you have allowed your body image to lead your choices, relationships, desires, and more. Your body and soul have dictated your identity. But that is about to change FOREVER.

To get the most out of this program, you will need to tell the OLD YOU, the "body-focused YOU", that it is on a serious and indefinite TIME OUT and will no longer rule your consciousness. Your goal over the next few weeks will be to silence it and let God's Spirit take over. Eventually, you will be transformed by the renewing of your mind and separate yourself from its ways of thinking, living, eating, and behaving.

P. **PAUSE and consider where the voices in your mind are coming from. Are they aligned with truth, or are they echoes of fear, shame, and old conditioning?**

"... we take captive every thought to make it obedient to Christ."
— 2 Corinthians 10:5

R. **REFLECT on the people, environments, and influences shaping your thoughts and emotions.**

"Set your minds on things above, not on earthly things.
For you died, and your life is now hidden with Christ in God."
— Colossians 3:2-3

A. **ASK the Holy Spirit what His thoughts are for you and how He wants you to live.**

"If any of you lacks wisdom, let him ask of God, who gives to all liberally
and without reproach, and it will be given to him."
— James 1:5

Y. **YIELD and obey what the Holy Spirit asks of you, no matter how difficult it may seem.**

"Listen! Obedience is better than sacrifice."
— 1 Samuel 15:22

As you learn to P.R.A.Y., you will also learn to STAND FIRM in this new life by putting on the full Armor of God each day.

"Stand therefore, having girded your waist with truth, having put on the breastplate of righteousness, and having shod your feet with the preparation of the gospel of peace; above all, taking the shield of faith with which you will be able to quench all the fiery darts of the wicked one. And take the helmet of salvation, and the sword of the Spirit, which is the word of God."
— Ephesians 6:14-17

In Biblical times, armor served as a crucial defense strategy, safeguarding the physical body and protecting vital organs from external threats. In the same way, the spiritual armor God provides protects your mind, emotions, and identity from the enemy's lies.

When feelings of fear, anger, confusion, anxiety, or despair begin to rise, it is often a signal that a piece of that armor has been neglected.

Truth protects your mind.
Righteousness guards your heart.
Faith shields you from attack.
Salvation anchors your identity.
And the Word of God becomes your weapon.

Whether it is the helmet of your salvation, the breastplate of your right-standing with God, or the belt of truth, the armor God gives you is your protection from the enemy's lies that come to kill, steal, and destroy your victory.

When fully armored with the spiritual defenses God provides, you stand with confidence, peace, and authority, unshaken by the forces around you.

The Apostle Paul understood the reality of spiritual warfare. Having personally endured persecution, imprisonment, and opposition, he urged believers to clothe themselves in God's protection.

"Therefore put on the full armor of God, so that when the day of evil comes, you may be able to stand your ground, and after you have done everything, to stand. Stand firm then, with the belt of truth buckled around your waist."
— Ephesians 6:13–14

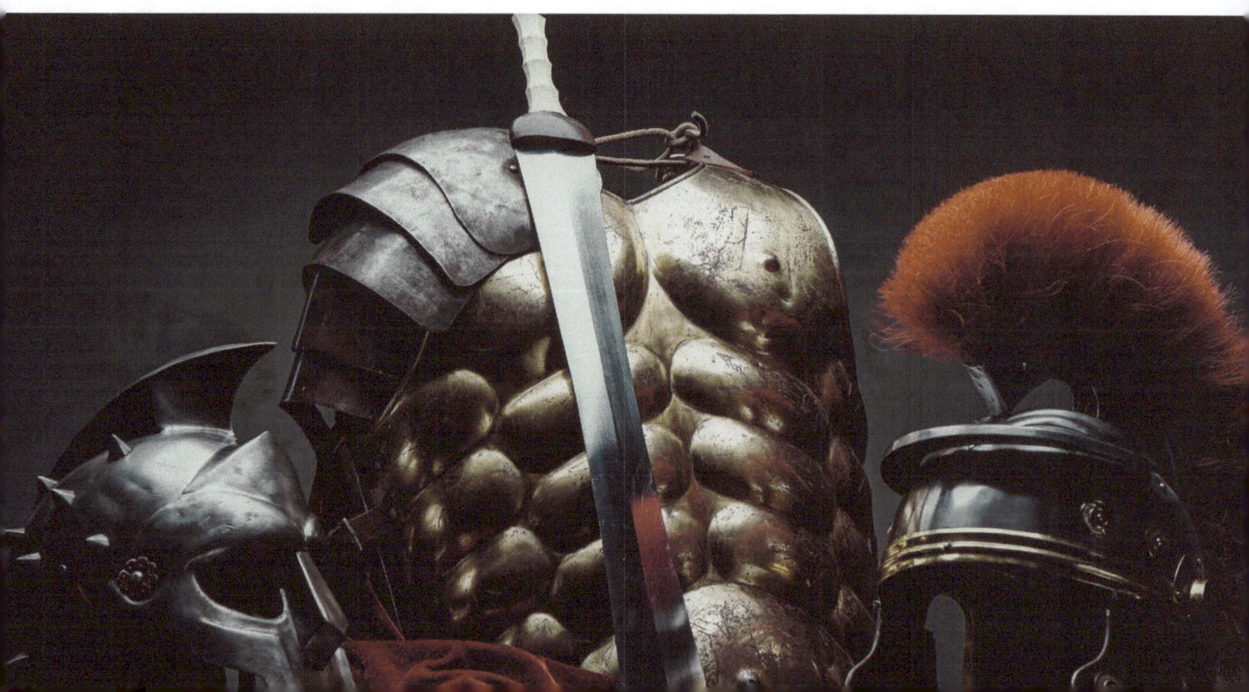

FUEL INTAKE

Document everything you eat this week, including breakfast, lunch, dinner, snacks, drinks, and candies. Do not change your eating habits this week so we have a clear baseline of your current behaviors.

DAY ONE:
DAY TWO:
DAY THREE:
DAY FOUR:
DAY FIVE:
DAY SIX:
DAY SEVEN:

PILLAR 3:
HYDRATION

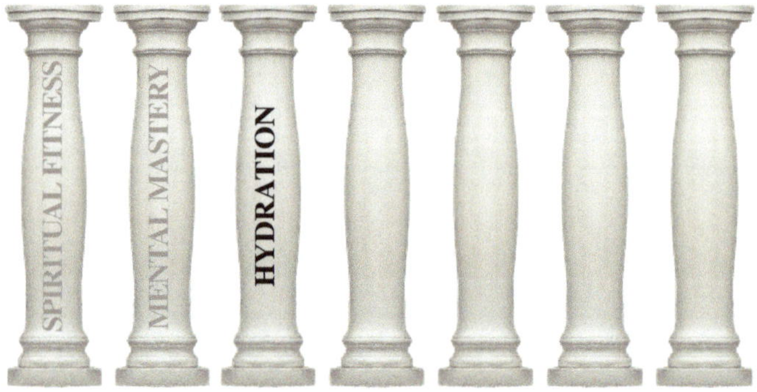

"You will be like a well-watered garden,
like a spring whose waters never fail."
— Isaiah 58:11

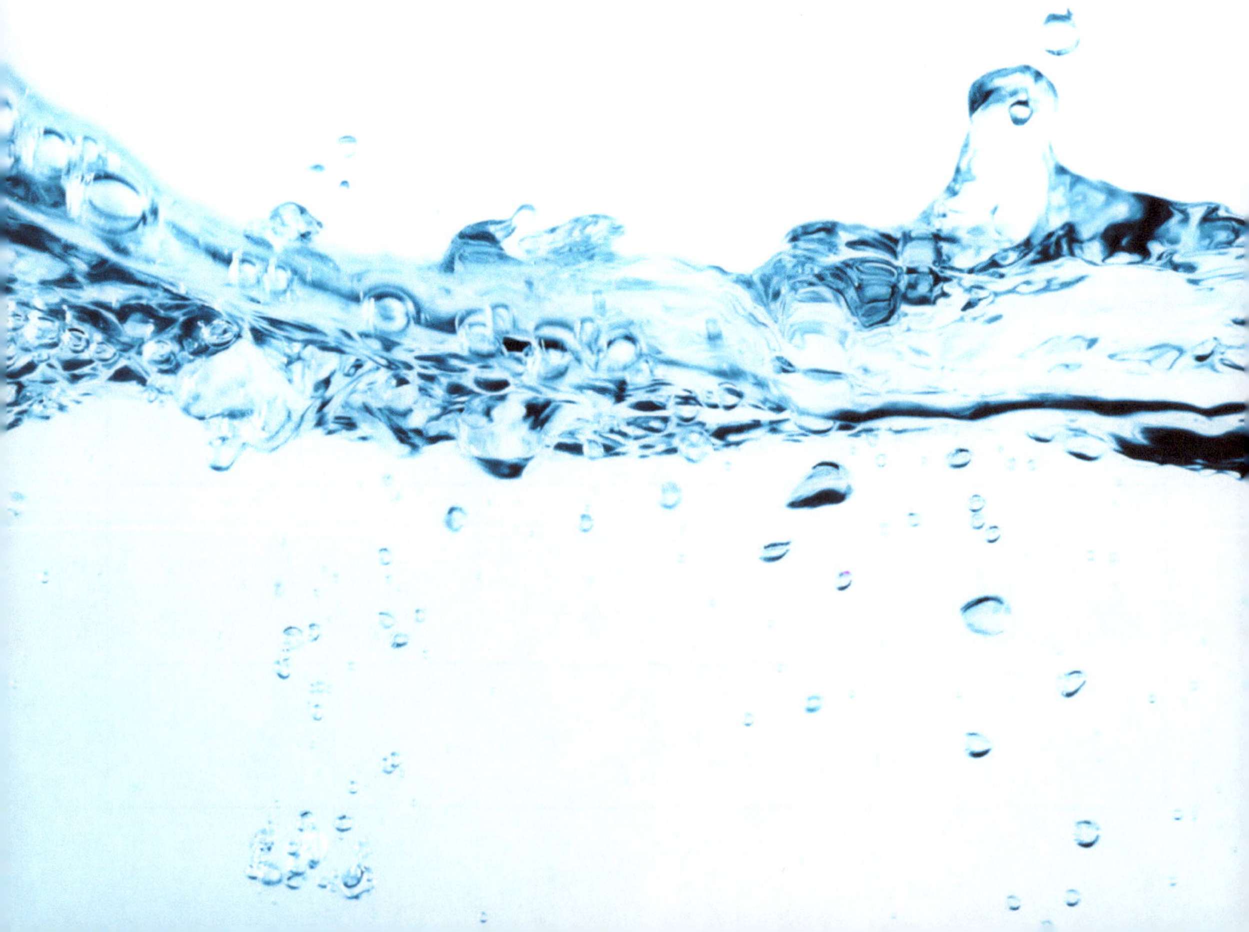

CHAPTER 3

STREAMS IN THE DESERT

Imagine being stranded in the desert. The sun is relentless. The air is dry. Your mouth becomes parched, your lips begin to crack, and your energy slowly drains. At first, you feel uncomfortable. Then your body grows weak. Soon, a migraine penetrates your head, and suddenly your body begins to shut down.

In that moment of dehydration and physical collapse, nothing else matters. Not success. Not money. Not another sale. Not entertainment. Only one thing matters.

Water.

There is a reason Scripture repeatedly uses water as a metaphor for life itself. As the Israelites wandered in the wilderness, they quickly discovered that without water, they would perish. In Exodus 17, the people were crying out in desperation when God instructed Moses to strike the rock. As he did so, water flowed like a stream in the middle of the desert, sustaining an entire nation.

God was teaching them something profound. **Both water and life flow from the hand of God.**

Centuries later, Jesus stood before a thirsty crowd and declared:

"If anyone thirsts, let him come to Me and drink."
— John 7:37

God designed the body to function with a critical need for water. Much like the body can't survive without water, the human spirit cannot thrive without the river of life that comes from God.

David understood this connection when he wrote:

"My soul thirsts for You, my flesh longs for You
in a dry and weary land where there is no water."
— Psalm 63:1

Throughout Scripture, water represents renewal, cleansing, and life.

The prophet Isaiah declared:

"You will be like a well-watered garden, like a spring whose waters never fail."
— Isaiah 58:11

From the beginning of creation, God designed water to sustain life. Every cell in your body depends on it. Every organ relies on it. Without it, life begins to break down. And like water, your spirit was designed to live in the presence of the One who called Himself Living Water.

"Whoever drinks the water I give them will never thirst. Indeed, the water I give them will become in them a spring of water welling up to eternal life."
— John 4:14

THE ULTIMATE LIFE SOURCE

In Genesis 1:2, we see the Spirit of God hovering over the waters.

Imagine the Creator looking upon those waters the way a master potter studies clay before shaping it and asking, "What shall we create today?"

From the very beginning of creation, water was central to life. Water is the single most important nutrient your body receives. It makes up more than sixty percent of your physical structure. While the human body can survive several weeks without food, most people can only survive three to five days without water. Every cell, organ, and system in your body depends on it.

Consider the extraordinary design of the human body. Your brain contains millions of pain receptors and hundreds of thousands of sensory detectors. Your eyes contain more than one hundred million light receptors that allow you to see with remarkable clarity. Your ears contain thousands of delicate fibers that vibrate to produce sound.

Your body contains more than 500 muscles, 200 bones, and approximately seven miles of nerve fibers. Your heart beats over 36 million times each year, pumping blood through more than 60,000 miles of veins and capillaries. Every one of these systems relies on proper hydration. Water is not simply something you drink. It is the environment in which life functions.

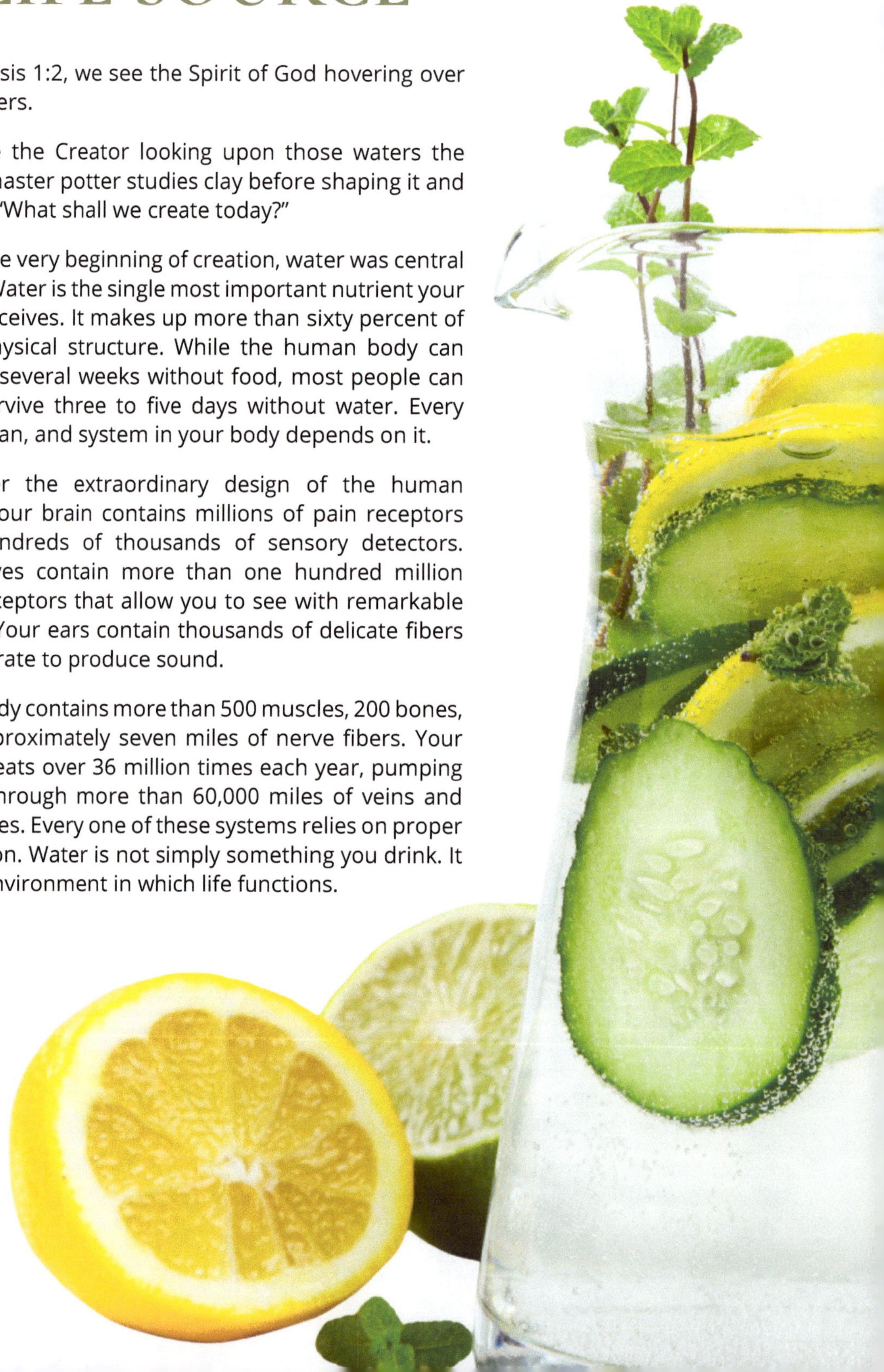

The secret is in the NUMBERS

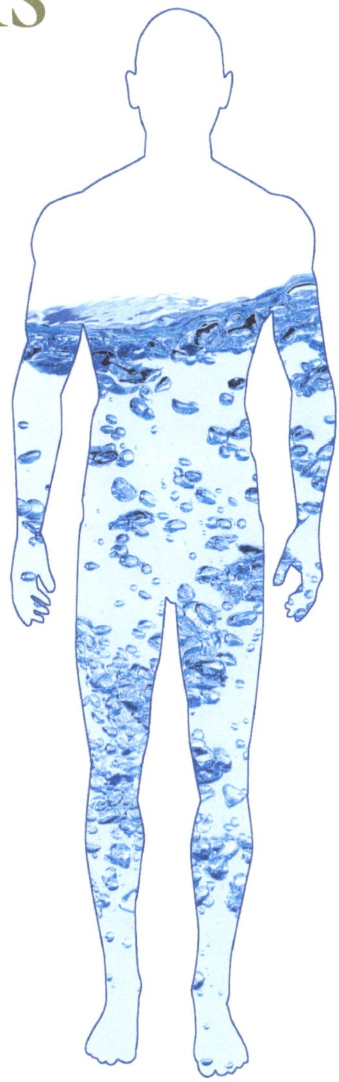

Why is water essential to optimal wellness? Because most of the human body is made of water. According to research published in the *Journal of Biological Chemistry,* many of the body's most vital organs are primarily composed of water.

Eyes - **95% water**
Brain - **83% water**
Lungs - **83% water**
Muscles - **79% water**
Heart - **73% water**
Kidneys - **83% water**
Skin - **64% water**

Your body is constantly signaling when hydration levels begin to drop. These signals often appear as symptoms:

Headaches
Muscle cramps
Joint pain
Migraines
Skin problems
Digestive issues
Fatigue

Before assuming something is seriously wrong, it may simply be your body asking for water.

Just as a car's dashboard warning light alerts you when fuel is low, your body sends signals when hydration levels drop.

Before reaching for medication, try rehydrating your body with clean water and observe how it responds.

Dehydration Test - True or False

- Headaches are a sign of dehydration. ________
- Muscle cramps could be a sign of dehydration. ________
- Your body doesn't need as much water in cold weather as in warm weather. ________
- Coffee can help you achieve your recommended intake of water each day. ________
- The body loses as much water when asleep as when awake. ________
- Your body loses hydration only through urine elimination. ________

*Answers - T, T, F, F, T, F

"For I will pour water on the thirsty land, and streams on the dry ground; I will pour my Spirit upon your offspring, and my blessing on your descendants."
— Isaiah 44:3

THE ANSWER

Before we were married, my husband Larry was an elite bodybuilder and a passionate advocate for hydration. Whenever I mentioned a headache, he would ask the same question.

"Have you been drinking enough water today?"

If I complained about cramps or muscle soreness, he would ask again. "Have you been drinking enough water?"

If I said I felt tired or nauseous, he would repeat the same question. Eventually, it started to sound like a broken record. So I decided to do my own research, and to my surprise, he was right.

My body was not craving medication. It was craving water. The headaches, cramps, and fatigue were often signals that my body simply needed hydration. Pure, clean water.

And if that alone does not convince you, here is something even more compelling. Proper hydration can slow many visible signs of aging and can significantly support weight loss. Sometimes the most powerful health solution is also the simplest. Water.

Interesting Facts:

Your body is made up of about 60-70% water. Your brain cells are about 80% water. Water increases the efficiency of your immune system.

Water helps reduce the risk of clogging of the arteries by reducing blood viscosity, improving the blood flow, and maintaining the integrity of the blood vessels.

Research shows that hydration affects brain function and cognition, especially in children and the elderly, and during exertion or heat exposure. Even mild dehydration can impair attention, memory, and mood, which are often symptoms of ADD, asthma, and other illnesses.

Alarming Facts:

The majority of all Americans are highly dehydrated. Often symptoms of disease are the first signal of your body needing more water. Your body loses about 2 quarts of water a day through perspiration, urination, and exhalation.

Water dehydration = painful symptoms

Good News... instead of giving up on living a life of vitality and wellness, start with the core fundamental to nutrition and that is to boost your water supply. Water, very well, could be your miracle cure!

How Much Water Is ENOUGH WATER?

Drinking enough water is essential to supporting a life of divine health.

So how much is enough?

One of the simplest ways to calculate your daily water intake is to drink half of your body weight in ounces each day.

If you weigh 140 pounds, aim for approximately 70 ounces of water daily.
If you weigh 200 pounds, aim for around 100 ounces.

For many people, this number is higher than what they are currently drinking. And much like a gurgling engine out of gas, your body will tell you when something is missing by sending off signals or symptoms.

Fatigue, headaches, digestive discomfort, muscle cramps, brain fog and dry skin are just a few signals your body is communicating with. And hydration is one of the simplest ways to support nearly every system in your body.

Later in this book we will explore the quality of water and how different types can influence your health.

For now, begin by increasing
your daily intake of clean water.

Your body will thank you.

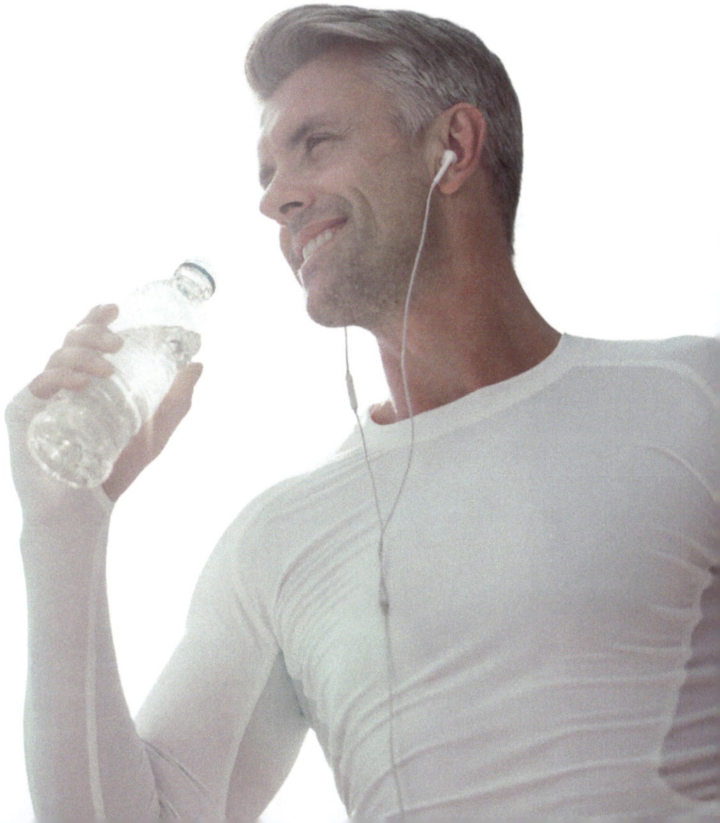

When Should I Drink WATER?

While hydration is essential for health, when and how you drink water can significantly impact digestion and nutrient absorption.

Drinking large amounts of water during meals can dilute stomach acid, which plays a very important role in digestion.

Stomach acid typically maintains a pH between 1 and 3 and helps break down food efficiently. When large amounts of water are consumed during meals, digestion may slow and food may remain in the stomach longer than necessary. This may reduce nutrient absorption and potentially lead to food sensitivities.

To promote optimal digestive health and ensure effective nutrient uptake, it is best to drink water before meals or wait an hour after eating. This practice helps maintain the acidic environment your stomach needs to digest food properly.

To support healthy digestion, consider these guidelines.

Upon Waking:
Drink a large glass of water to rehydrate your body after a night of sleep and help activate your metabolism.

Between Meals:
Drinking water thirty minutes before meals can support hydration and digestion.

During Meals:
Limit water intake to small sips if needed.

Before Sleep:
A small glass of water can help maintain hydration overnight, though you may initially notice increased nighttime bathroom visits as your body adjusts.

These small adjustments can improve digestion, hydration, and overall wellness.

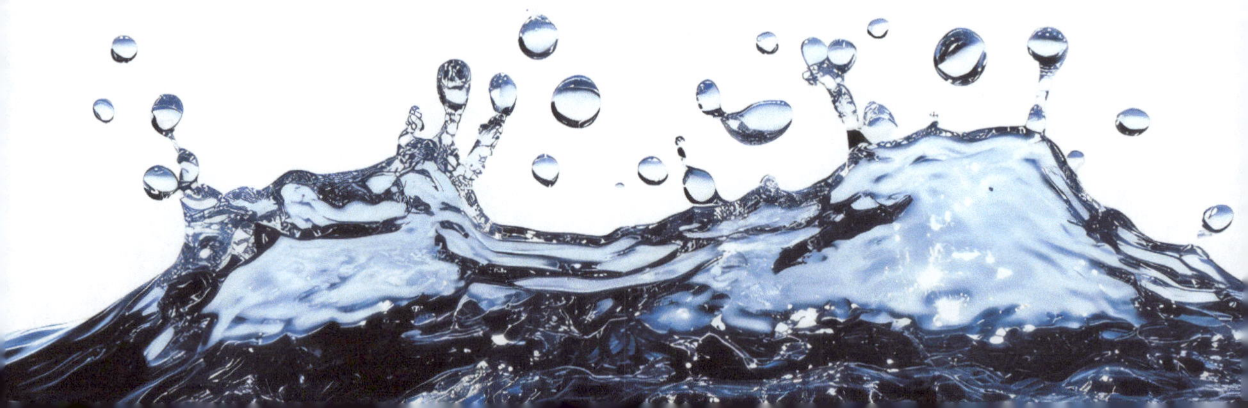

WHICH TYPE OF WATER should I drink?

Not all water is equal. Different types of water can affect the body in different ways.

1. **Alkaline Water:** With a higher pH level than regular drinking water, alkaline water may help neutralize excess acidity in the body.
2. **Hydrogen Water:** This water is infused with additional hydrogen molecules. Research suggests it can increase energy, improve recovery after workouts, improve gut health, and reduce inflammation by offering antioxidant properties that fight free radicals.
3. **Alkaline Ionized Water:** Similar to alkaline water but created using an ionizer, this water also offers antioxidant properties due to its negative oxidation-reduction potential (ORP). It is said to enhance digestion, metabolic health and detox effects.
4. **Reverse Osmosis Water:** This purification process removes contaminants and impurities, including toxins, bacteria, and heavy metals. However, it also strips away beneficial minerals, so they often need to be reintroduced into the water.
5. **Distilled Water:** The purest form of water, distilled water has had all its minerals and impurities removed through boiling and condensation. However, its lack of minerals can make it less ideal for drinking, as it may cause mineral depletion in the body over time.

Knowing these differences is key, as each type impacts the body uniquely, influencing everything from your energy levels to how effectively your body can absorb and utilize the water you drink. Choose wisely based on your health needs and the quality of water you have access to. And if you want to add a little pizzazz to your water, try infusing it with fresh lime, orange, mint, lemon or strawberries.

The best option often depends on your health goals and the quality of water available to you.

Consistent hydration can dramatically influence your energy levels, mental clarity, skin health, and overall vitality.

Sometimes the simplest habit creates the greatest transformation.

Drink more water.

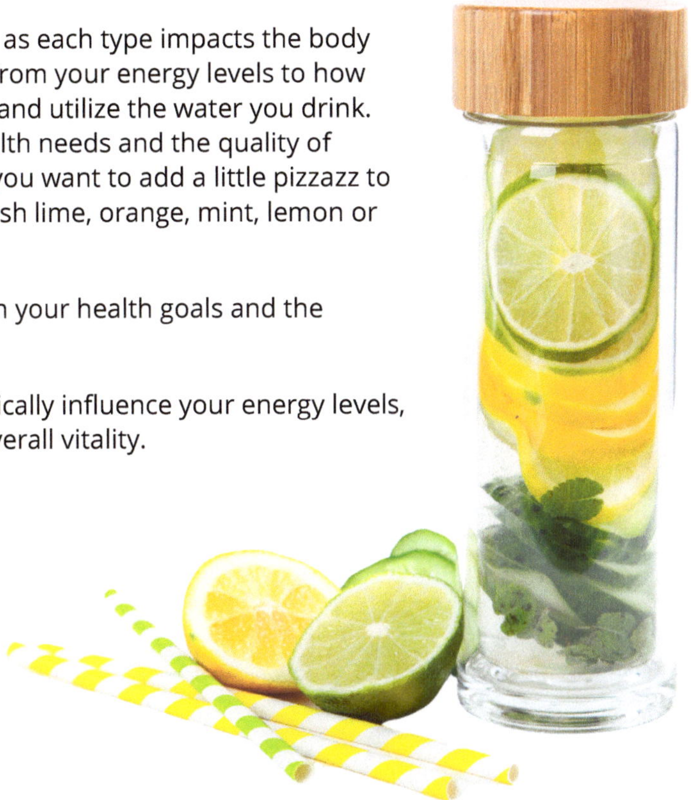

PILLAR 4: NUTRITION

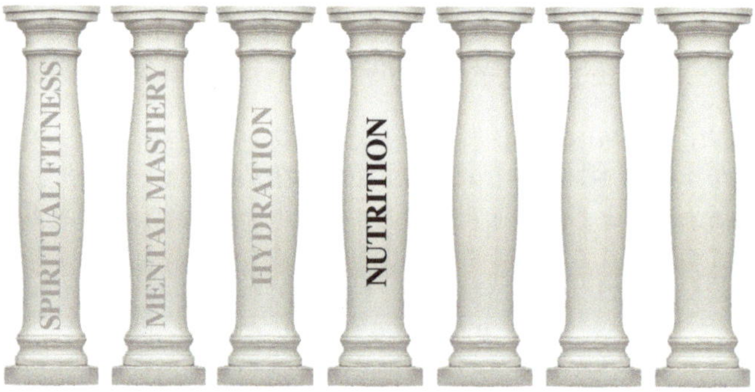

"Then God said, 'I give you every seed-bearing plant on the face of the whole earth and every tree that has fruit with seed in it. They will be yours for food'."
— Genesis 1:29

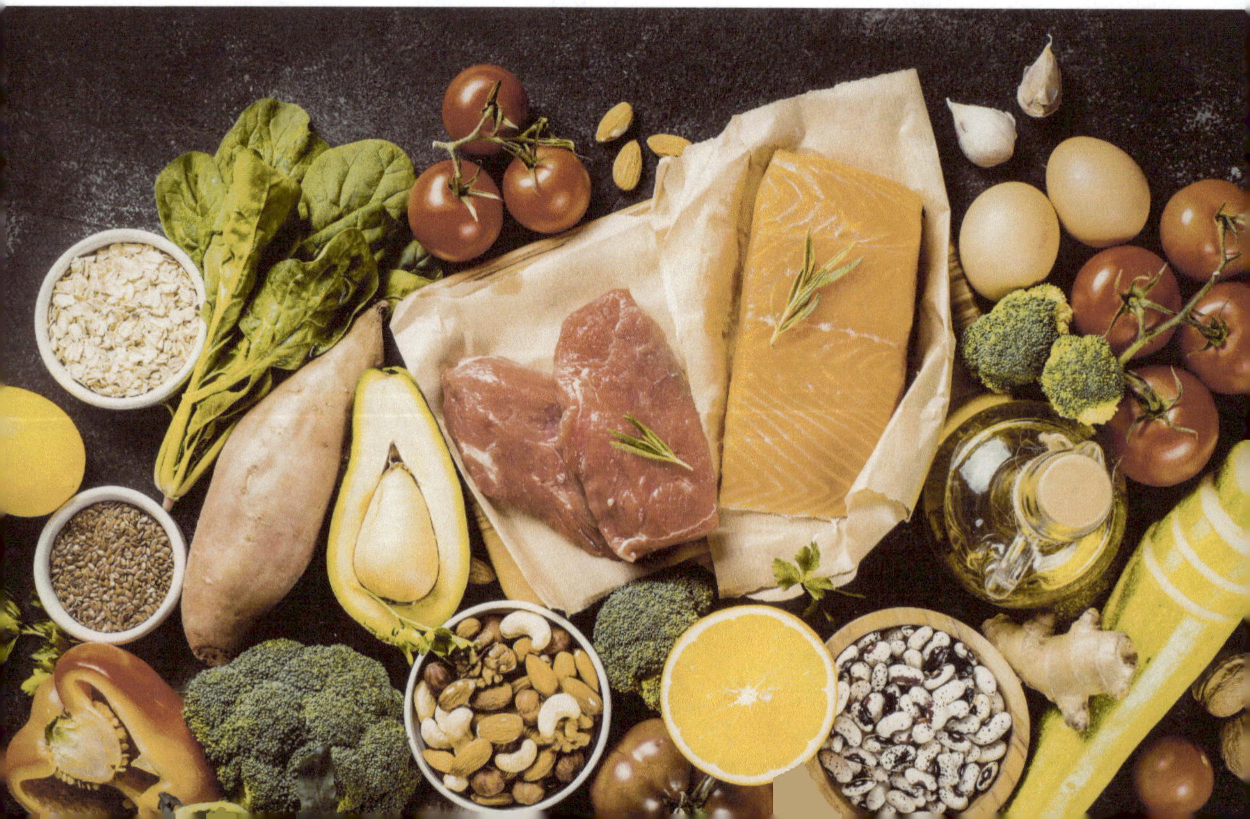

CHAPTER 4

FOOD IS FUEL

From the beginning of creation, God designed food and water to sustain life.

We see in Genesis that God provides mankind with every seed-bearing plant and fruit from the trees as nourishment. Food was not created to be emotional relief or entertainment. It was created as fuel. Yet somewhere along the way, our relationship with food changed.

Food became a celebration, a comfort, an emotional reward, and even an escape. Instead of fueling our bodies, we began feeding our emotions. This shift has had enormous consequences.

Today, our grocery stores are filled with artificial foods engineered to satiate cravings temporarily rather than nourish the body. Highly processed foods are manufactured to override the brain's natural appetite signals, leaving people feeling hungry even when their bodies have consumed more than enough calories.

The result is that we have become a culture that is overfed yet undernourished.

We eat more food than any generation in history. Let that sink in. Despite increased consumption, we struggle with fatigue, inflammation, joint issues, weight gain, and chronic disease at unprecedented levels.

The issue is not simply how much we eat. It is what we eat.
And just as importantly, why we eat it and when.

Your body is an extraordinary system designed by God to heal itself, repair itself, renew itself, and function with remarkable efficiency when given the proper fuel.

When you begin fueling your body with the nutrients it was designed to receive, something remarkable happens. Energy increases. Inflammation decreases. Mental clarity improves. And the body begins to move back toward its natural state of health.

Nutrition is not about restriction. It is about restoration.

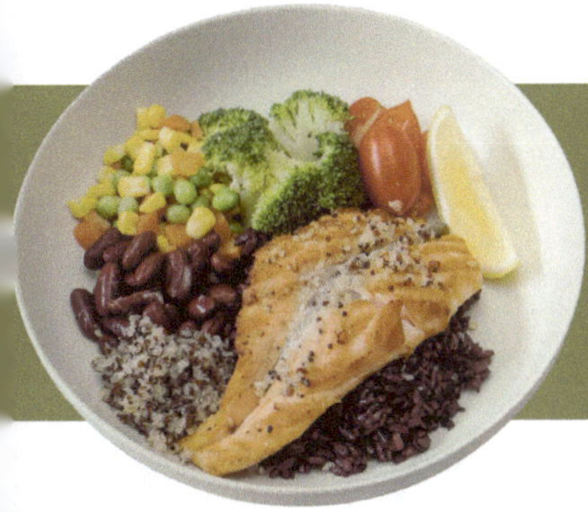

"Do you not know that your bodies are temples of the Holy Spirit, who is in you, whom you have received from God? You are not your own; you were bought at a price. Therefore honor God with your bodies."
— 1 Corinthians 6:19-20

THE GARDEN VS THE LAB

From the very beginning of time, God defined what food was meant to be.

He laid out the perfect meal plan in the Garden of Eden where nourishment came directly from creation. He gave us seeds, plants, fruit, and living food filled with life, energy, and nutrition. Nothing was engineered. Nothing was synthetic. Nothing required a factory. Food came from the ground that God created. It was simple. It was living. And it sustained life.

Today, however, much of what fills the shelves in grocery stores no longer resembles what God first gave us. Instead of seeds and plants, we have highly processed, manufactured foods created in laboratories and factories.

Colors are injected. Flavors are engineered. Shelf life is extended with chemicals. And nutrients have been stripped away in the hopes of creating long-lasting, money-generating products that drive marketplace excitement.

We have slowly moved from the garden to the laboratory. This is why returning to God's design for food is not just a health decision. It's stewardship.

Think of nutrition like climbing a ladder.

At the bottom of the ladder are all of the engineered and highly addictive foods, pills, and artificial products that fill us up but leave us starving for nutrition. Each step up the ladder brings you closer to foods that carry life and health. Each step downward moves toward foods that are increasingly artificial and destructive.

The goal is not perfection.
The goal is progress.
Every meal is an opportunity to climb higher.

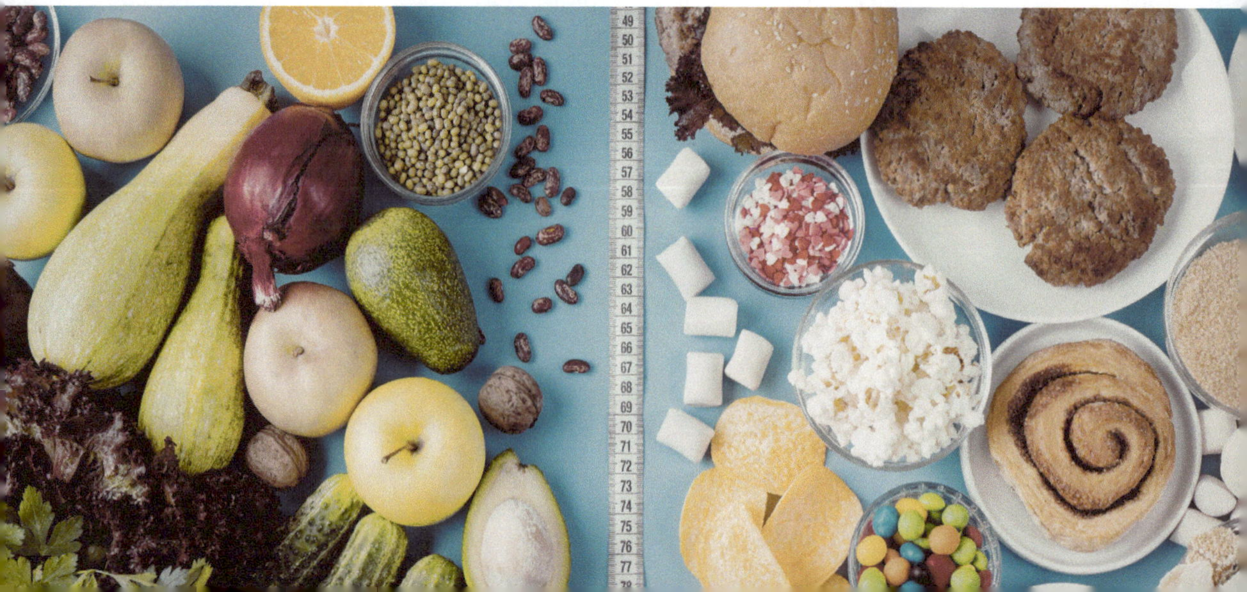

THE LADDER OF LIFE

Moving from man-made food to God-made fuel

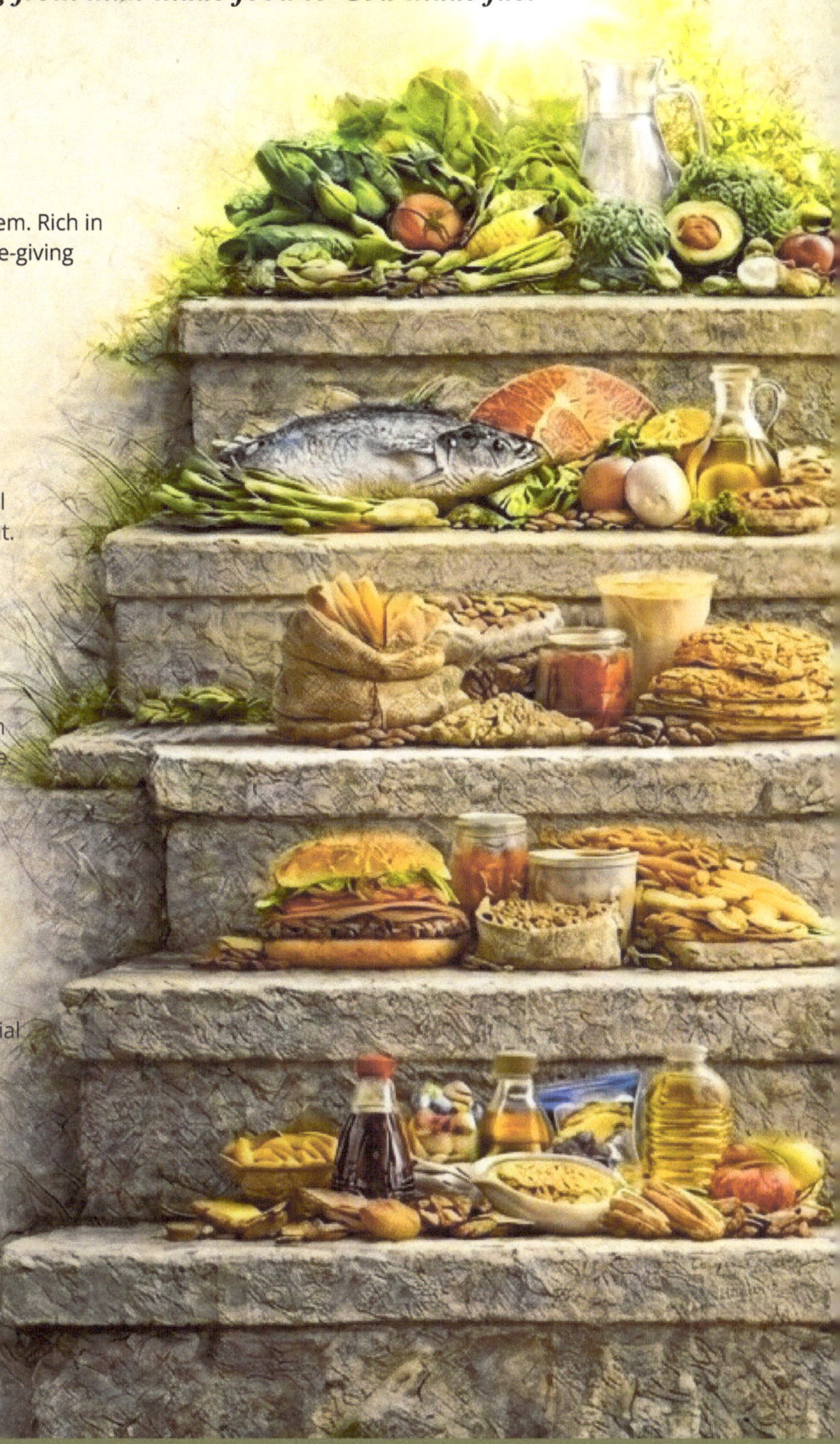

LEVEL 5

LIVING FOODS

Foods closest to how God created them. Rich in enzymes, minerals, hydration, and life-giving nutrients (Genesis 1:29)

LEVEL 4

WHOLE FOODS

Foods that still resemble their natural form and provide strong nourishment.

LEVEL 3

PROCESSED FOODS

Foods altered from their natural form that contain reduced nutritional value.

LEVEL 2

ULTRA-PROCESSED FOOD

Foods engineered for taste and shelf life rather than nourishment. Industrial formulations with many chemical ingredients.

LEVEL 1

CHEMICAL FOODS

Artificial colorings, flavors, synthetic sweeteners, and non-food additives engineered in laboratories.

Progress Over Perfection

The higher you climb, the more life your body receives.

ELEVATE YOUR CHOICES
ELEVATE YOUR LIFE

Today, most people unknowingly live on the lower half of the ladder.

The modern diet is dominated by ultra-processed foods that were never part of God's original design. As these foods became more common, something else began to rise with them.

The goal is not perfection.
The goal is progress.
Every meal is an opportunity to climb higher.

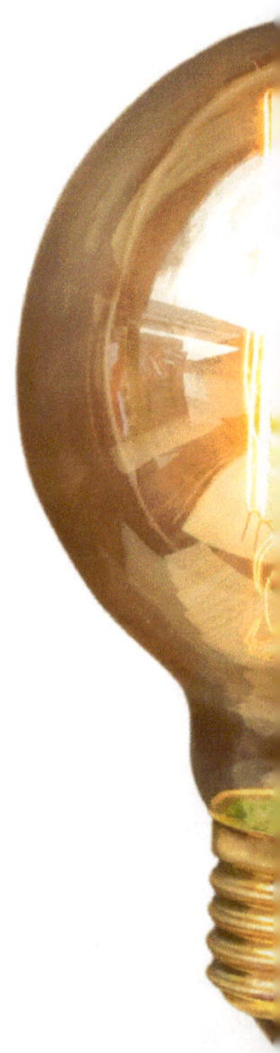

The world today is saturated with chronic illness. Fatigue, inflammation, joint pain, metabolic disorders, cardiovascular disease, and autoimmune conditions have become common realities for millions of people.

Yet the human body was never designed for a life of constant sickness.

God created the human body with extraordinary systems of healing, repair, and renewal. When properly fueled, the body has an incredible ability to restore balance and maintain health.

So the question becomes simple.

If the body was designed for health, why are so many people sick?

Elevate Your Thinking... Elevate Your Choices

Health is rarely transformed through one dramatic decision.
It is shaped by the small choices we repeat every day.

Every meal is an opportunity to move one step higher.

Choose foods that nourish your body. Choose habits that support life.
Choose the path that leads upward.

Because the higher you climb, the more life your body receives and the more vitality you have to give to the things and people who matter most.

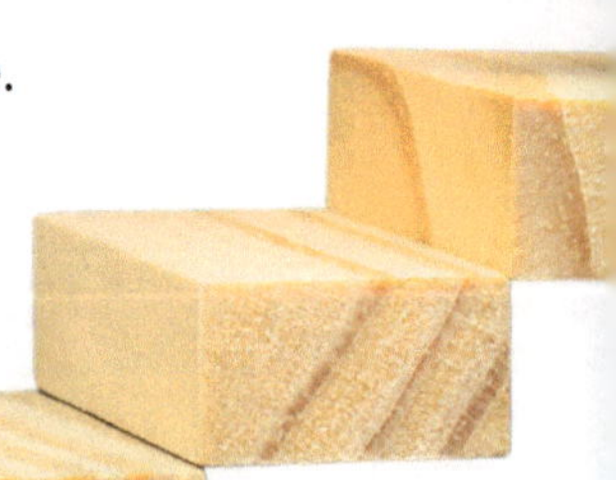

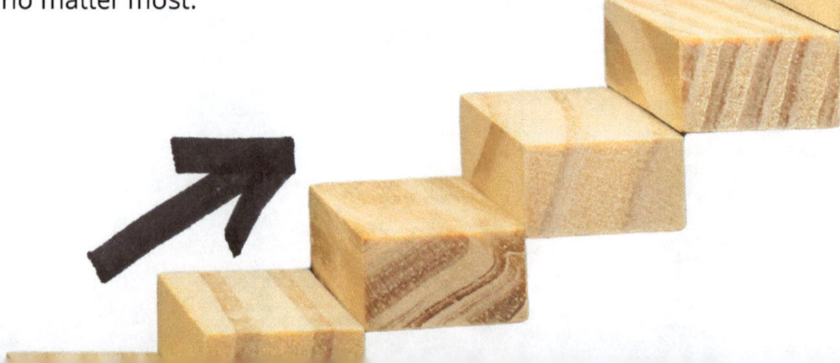

CHAPTER 5

ACID OVERLOAD

Your Body Is Always Talking

When the body is properly nourished and hydrated, it has an extraordinary ability to maintain equilibrium. But when acid-forming inputs overwhelm the system, the body is forced into constant correction mode.

One major contributor to modern illness is something most people rarely consider: acid overload.

Imagine a car battery that becomes damaged when acid builds up and begins to corrode its internal components. Something similar can occur within the body when acidic waste accumulates faster than the body can neutralize or eliminate it.

Excess acidity places stress on tissues and organs. It can contribute to inflammation, weakened bones, poor circulation, fatigue, hormonal imbalance, and long-term disease. The body works constantly to maintain balance. But when acid-forming foods dominate the diet, the body must work overtime to protect vital systems.

Over time, the body begins to pay the price.

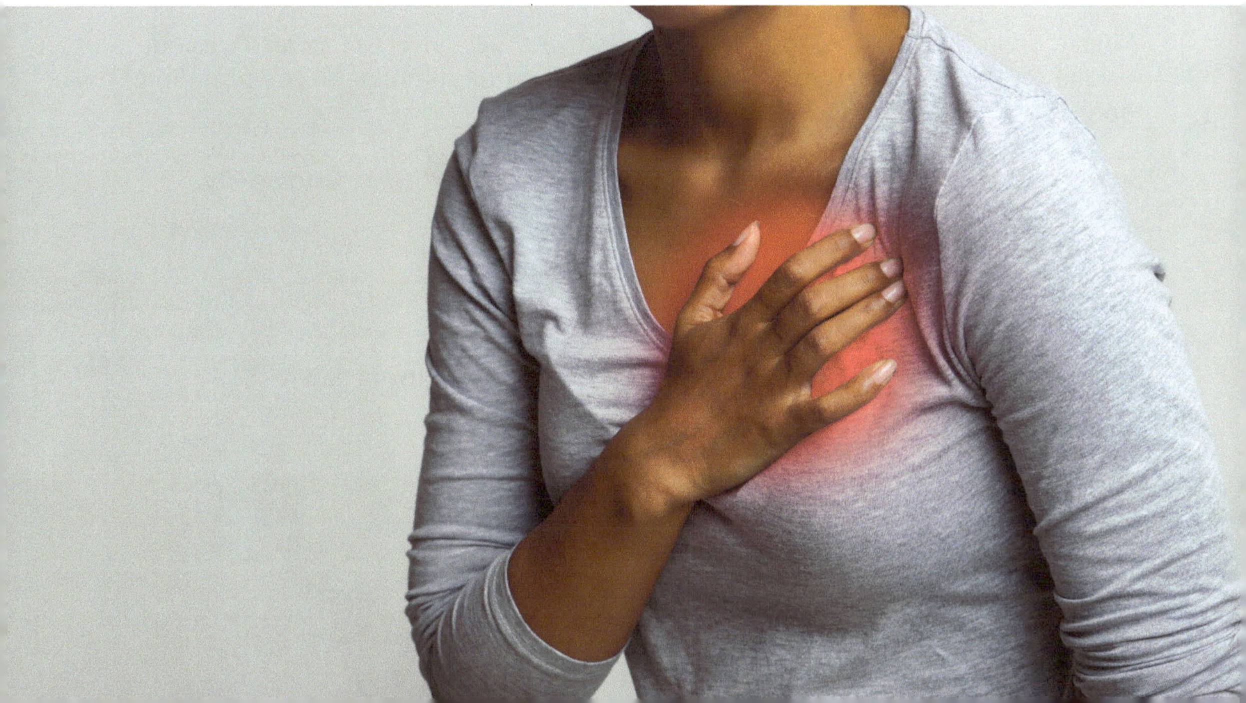

THE ROOT OF THE MATTER

So how did we get here? The answer is surprisingly simple. Three forces are quietly pushing modern culture toward acidity and disease.

Stress

Life in modern society is almost synonymous with stress. Deadlines, financial pressure, constant stimulation, and emotional strain all activate the body's stress response. When stress hormones remain elevated, the body produces more acidic waste, and inflammation begins to rise.

Dehydration

Nearly seventy percent of Americans live in a chronic state of dehydration. Water plays a critical role in flushing acids and toxins from the body. When hydration is low, waste accumulates, and the body struggles to maintain balance. Dehydration also weakens the body's ability to regulate hunger and metabolism.

Poor Diet

The modern diet is heavily dominated by processed foods that were never part of God's original design for nourishment. Instead of whole foods grown from the earth, many meals now come from factories and laboratories.

Highly refined grains, sugary drinks, fast food, and packaged snacks flood the body with acid- forming compounds while providing very little nutritional support.

Instead of consuming foods that restore balance, most people unknowingly fuel the very conditions that lead to illness.

Understanding this imbalance reveals why the quality of our food matters so much.

When food is digested, the body leaves behind what scientists call an "ash" residue. This residue can be acidic, neutral, or alkaline depending on the mineral composition of the food.

Some foods help restore balance. Others push the body further toward acidity.

The key to vibrant health is learning how to recognize the difference.

This brings us to an important question.

Is the food you eat building your health, or slowly breaking it down?

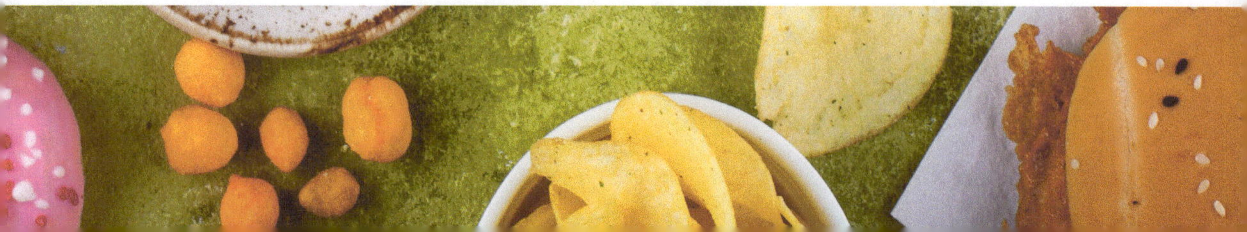

YOUR BODY ISN'T BROKEN IT'S RESPONDING

For many people, symptoms feel frightening. A fever spikes. A rash appears. Fatigue sets in. A child begins coughing through the night. The immediate assumption is that something is wrong.

But what if the body is not failing? What if it is responding?

Your body is one of the most brilliantly designed systems on Earth. Every organ, cell, and hormone is constantly working to protect you and maintain balance. When toxins enter the body, it attempts to eliminate them. When inflammation rises, repair systems activate. When nutrients are lacking, the body slows certain processes in order to conserve energy.

What many people call disease is often the body sounding an alarm. It is communicating. And sometimes the most important thing we can do is pause long enough to listen. I learned this lesson early on as a young mother.

When our children were young, long before functional wellness and alternative approaches became more widely accepted, many of our choices were questioned.

When the world rushed toward certain medical practices, Larry and I paused. We studied. We prayed. We asked questions about what we were being asked to put into our children's bodies. Sometimes that meant choosing a different path than most families around us.

It wasn't always popular.

Even though we homeschooled our children for most of their education, there were three years when they attended a private Christian school. Every year I was asked to sign exemption forms acknowledging that our family had chosen a different approach to certain medical procedures.

Some people assumed we were reckless. But our motivation was simple. We believed God designed the human body with extraordinary intelligence. And we wanted to learn how that design worked. As a result, our children were rarely sick. When colds or flu moved through the community, their immune systems often fought the illness quickly.

One moment in particular shaped our understanding forever.

Our son, Payton, was about six years old when he brought home a friend from school who clearly had a nasty cold. The boy had a green runny nose and obvious symptoms of illness. Within a couple of days, Payton began showing similar symptoms. His fever quickly rose to over 103 degrees.

Many parents would have immediately rushed to medication or the doctor. But I had begun learning something about the body. A fever is not the enemy. It is one of the body's most powerful defense mechanisms. The increase in temperature helps the immune system fight viruses and bacteria.

Instead of panicking, we supported his body. We cooled him with lukewarm baths, placed cool towels on his forehead, prayed, and allowed the fever to do what it was designed to do. Within a short time, his body fought off the illness. Our knowledge bank was filled, and little did we know that every little sickness or setback was a setup for us to gain resilience in our faith.

Another experience taught us an even deeper lesson.

At one point, our baby daughter began having a runny nose seemingly out of nowhere. At the time, I was traveling on tour with Zig Ziglar and several other world leaders. I had taken her with me while our son stayed home with a nanny. As her nose continued running and she became increasingly fussy, I decided to take her to a clinic just to have her ears checked before our flight. I wanted to make sure the altitude wouldn't cause problems.

But when the doctors examined her, the atmosphere in the room suddenly changed. They rushed her out for emergency tests. My heart dropped. I was alone. Larry was in Japan on business. My family lived hours away.

When they returned fifteen minutes later, they told me they wanted to perform a spinal tap to rule out bacterial meningitis. My legs nearly gave out. I had only come in to check her ears.

I called Larry in tears. "Honey, they want to do a spinal tap. This feels extreme. I have no peace about it." We were young parents. We were not doctors. But we believed in prayer.

Larry stopped everything and prayed for wisdom. When he finished, he said something I will never forget.

"Honey, I'm not there to discern the moment. You're going to have to listen to what the Holy Spirit is telling you to do. I trust you."

I told the doctors I wanted to wait twenty-four hours before agreeing to such an invasive procedure.

They strongly disagreed.

Eventually, they brought legal documents into the room, releasing them from liability for any harm that might come to my daughter if I refused their recommendation.

I was thirty-one years old, scared, and completely alone. But I signed the papers and left the clinic. Not out of rebellion toward doctors. But because I had learned something important.

Wisdom often requires slowing down long enough to listen.

That night I prayed and waited.

The next morning I woke to the sound of my baby crying again. When I went into her room, she had her hand in her mouth and tears running down her cheeks. As I gently pulled her hand away to comfort her, I felt something.

Her first tooth had broken through!

Her body wasn't broken. It was responding. What looked like a medical emergency was simply the natural process of teething.

That moment changed our perspective forever.

Over time Larry and I continued studying how the body works. We began to recognize that symptoms are often signals, not enemies.

The body communicates.

Fever can mean the immune system is fighting. Fatigue can mean the body is asking for rest. Inflammation can signal that something harmful has entered the system. Symptoms are not always the problem. Sometimes they are the body's attempt to solve the problem.

Which leads us to an important question.
What are we fueling our bodies with every day?
Because the foods we eat either supports the body's ability to heal or creates the very conditions that lead to disease.

And that brings us to an important principle in nutrition.

God gave us wisdom.
God gave us a garden.

When we begin to put the two together... we make better choices!

When we learn to listen to, nourish, and steward the body God created, we discover something remarkable. The body is designed to heal when it is properly fueled.

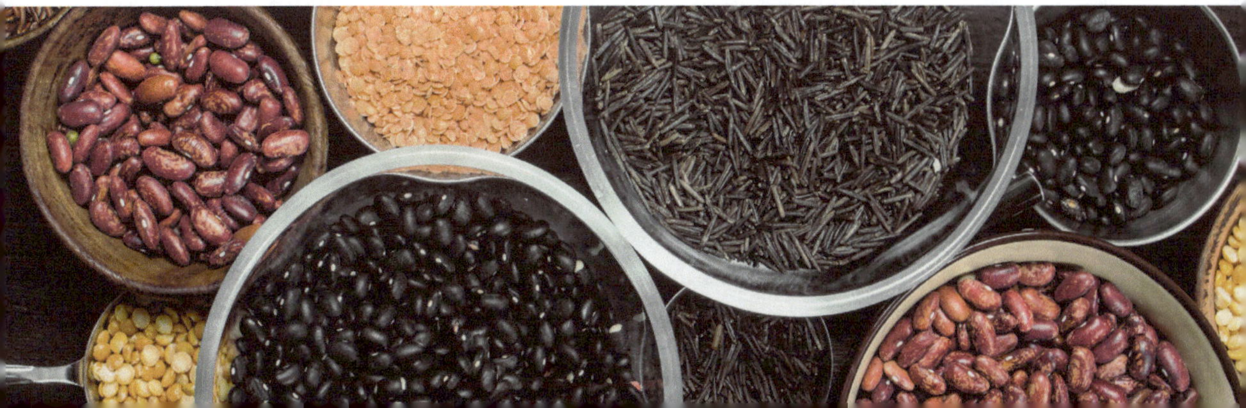

ACIDIC OR ALKALINE

Now that we know symptoms are not the enemy. How can we fuel our bodies for better outcomes? All food that enters the body is eventually broken down during digestion. It will either help or hurt the overall healing process. After this digestion, the body is left with what scientists call a metabolic "ash" residue. This residue can be acidic, neutral, or alkaline, depending largely on the mineral composition of the food.

For example, foods rich in minerals such as potassium, calcium, and magnesium tend to produce an alkaline effect in the body. Foods high in sulfur, phosphorus, and certain proteins tend to produce a more acidic effect.

While the body works hard to regulate and maintain a stable internal pH, the foods we eat will either support that balance or make the body work much harder to maintain it. Over time, this constant demand can place stress on tissues, bones, and metabolic systems.

This is why nutrition quality matters so deeply.

In his popular book, *Alkalize or Die*, Theodore A. Baroody, M.A., D.C., N.D., Ph.D., shook the scientific world by saying, *"The countless names of illnesses do not really matter. What does matter is that they all come from the same root cause... TOO MUCH ACID IN THE BODY!"* Fortunately for us, it is easy to categorize which foods leave which kind of ash.

Acid-Forming Foods:

In general, foods such as refined sugars, processed grains, alcohol, heavily processed meats, and artificial additives tend to create a more acid-forming effect in the body. When these foods dominate the diet, the body must work harder to maintain its internal balance.

Alkaline-Forming Foods:

Vegetables are among the most powerful alkaline-forming foods available. Leafy greens, cucumbers, avocados, peppers, and most vegetables help support the body's natural buffering systems. Fresh fruits, seeds, nuts, and certain whole grains also contribute valuable minerals that help restore balance. In general, foods that come directly from the earth and remain close to their natural state tend to support an alkaline environment.

To Maintain pH Balance (80/20 Rule):

To support a healthy pH balance in your blood and tissues, aim for a diet made up of roughly seventy to eighty percent alkaline-forming foods and no more than twenty to thirty percent acid-forming foods. Ideally, at least half of those alkaline foods should be fresh and raw.

Raw foods naturally retain higher levels of enzymes and nutrients that support digestion and metabolic balance. While cooking can reduce some of these nutrients, many cooked foods still provide valuable nourishment. Unlike the traditional food pyramid many of us grew up with, which tends to emphasize more acid-forming foods, this approach restores balance by focusing on whole foods that come directly from the earth.

This reference chart helps identify which foods tend to be more alkaline or more acid-forming. Each food is assigned a number representing its approximate potential acid or alkaline load in the body. A positive number indicates alkaline potential while a negative number indicates acid potential. These charts are designed as simple tools to help guide food choices. Remember that the goal is balance, not perfection.

ALKALINE FOODS

VEGETABLES

Brussels Sprouts +0.5
Broccoli +6.8
Peas, Ripe +0.5
Asparagus +1.3
Comfrey +1.5
Green Cabbage +2.0
Lettuce +2.2
Onion +3.0
Cauliflower +3.1
White Cabbage +3.3
Green Cabbage (winter) +4.0
Savoy Cabbage +4.5
Barley Grass +28.1
Lamb's Lettuce +4.8
Peas, Fresh +5.1
Zucchini +5.7
Red Cabbage +6.3
Rhubarb Stalks +6.3
Leeks (Bulbs) +7.2
Watercress +7.7
French Green Beans +11.2
Sorrel +11.5
Spinach +13.1
Dog Grass +22.6
Dandelion +22.7
Garlic +13.2
Celery +13.3
Cabbage Lettuce, Fresh +14.1
Endive, Fresh +14.5
Cayenne Pepper +18.8
Straw Grass +21.4
Shave Grass +21.7
Sprouted Radish Seeds +28.4
Sprouted Chia Seeds +28.5
Alfalfa Grass +29.3
Cucumber, Fresh +31.5
Wheat Grass +33.8
Soy Sprouts +29.5
Red Radish +16.7
Chives +8.3

ROOT VEGETABLES

White Radish (Spring) +3.1
Rutabaga +3.1
Summer Black Radish +39.4
Kohlrabi +5.1
Horseradish +6.8
Turnip +8.0
Carrot +9.5
Beet +11.3

FRUITS

Limes +8.2
Fresh Lemon +9.9
Tomato +13.6
Avocado +15.6

"My people are destroyed for lack of knowledge."
— Hosea 4:6

NON-STORED GRAINS

Buckwheat Groats +0.5
Spelt +0.5
Lentils +0.6
Soy Flour +2.5
Tofu +3.2
Lima Beans +12.0
Soybeans, Fresh +12.0
White Beans (Navy Beans) +12.1
Granulated Soy (Cooked Ground Soy Beans) +12.8
Soy Nuts (soaked and air dried) +26.5
Soy Lecithin (Pure) +38.0

SEEDS & GRAINS

Sesame Seeds +0.5
Cumin Seeds +1.1
Fennel Seeds +1.3
Flax Seed Oil +3.5
Flax Seeds +1.3
Caraway Seeds +2.3
Sunflower Seeds +5.4
Evening Primrose Oil +4.1
Pumpkin Seeds +5.6
Wheat Kernel +11.4
Almonds +3.6
Olive Oil +1.0

ACIDIC FOODS

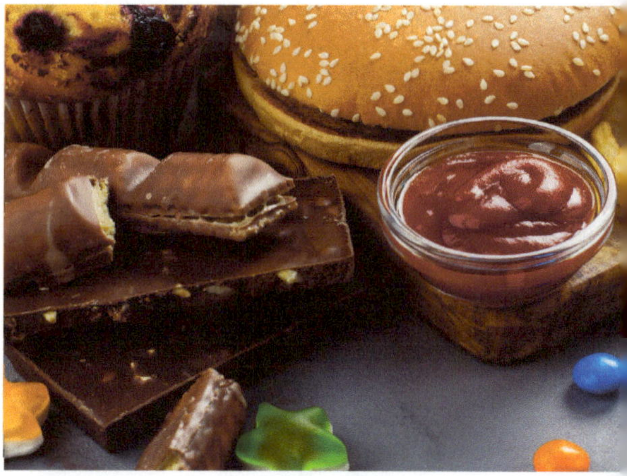

MEAT, POULTRY, AND FISH

Pork -38.0
Veal -35.0
Beef -34.5
Fresh Water Fish -11.8
Ocean Fish -20.0
Chicken -18.0
Eggs -22
Oysters -5.0
Liver -3.0
Organ Meats -3.0

FRUIT (CONSUME IN MODERATION)

Rose Hips -15.5
Pineapple -12.6
Mandarin Orange -11.5
Banana, Ripe -10.1
Pear -9.9
Peach -9.7
Cranberry -7.0
Black Currant -6.1
Fig Juice Powder -2.4
Apricot -9.5
Papaya -9.4
Orange -9.2
Mango -8.7
Tangerine -8.5
Currant -8.2
Gooseberry, Ripe -7.7
Strawberry -5.4
Blueberry -5.3
Raspberry -5.1
Yellow Plum -4.9
Italian Plum -4.9
Date -4.7
Grapefruit -1.7
Grape, Ripe -7.6
Date -4.7
Cherry, Sweet -3.6
Cherry, Sour +3.5
Banana, Unripe +4.8
Coconut, Fresh +0.5
Watermelon -1.0
Red Currant -2.4
Cantaloupe -2.5

DRINKS

Coffee -25.1
Liquor -38.7
Wine -16.4
Beer -26.8
Tea (Black) -27.1
Fruit Juice, Packaged, Natural -8.7
Fruit Juice Sweetened With White Sugar -33.6

CONDIMENTS

Ketchup -12.4
Mayonnaise -12.5
Mustard -19.2
Soy Sauce -36.2
Vinegar -39.4

BREADS

White Bread -10.0
White Biscuit -6.5
Whole-Meal Bread -6.5
Whole-Grain Bread -4.5
Brown Rice -12.5
Rye Bread -2.5
Wheat -10.1

NUTS

Walnuts -8.0
Pistachios -16.6
Macadamia Nuts -3.2
Peanuts -12.8
Hazelnuts -2.0
Cashews -9.3

MILK & DAIRY

According to Dr. Robert Young, who is an expert on the acid-alkaline balance, almost all dairy products (regular or low-fat) are major acid producers. As a result, the body must use up its resources of calcium (often leached from the bones and causing osteoporosis) and other minerals to neutralize these acids.

Hard Cheese -18.1
Quark -17.3
Cream -3.9
Homogenized Milk -1.0
Buttermilk +1.3

OTHER

Canned foods, microwaved foods, processed foods, alcohol, nicotine, as well as many prescription and over-the-counter drugs are also acid forming. If you are taking any prescriptions, it is very important to include lots of vegetables and other alkalizing foods in your diet to replenish your body's alkaline reserves, as well as getting enough sleep, exercise, clean water, and managing your stress.

CHAPTER 6

DEAD VS. LIVING FOODS

Choose life!

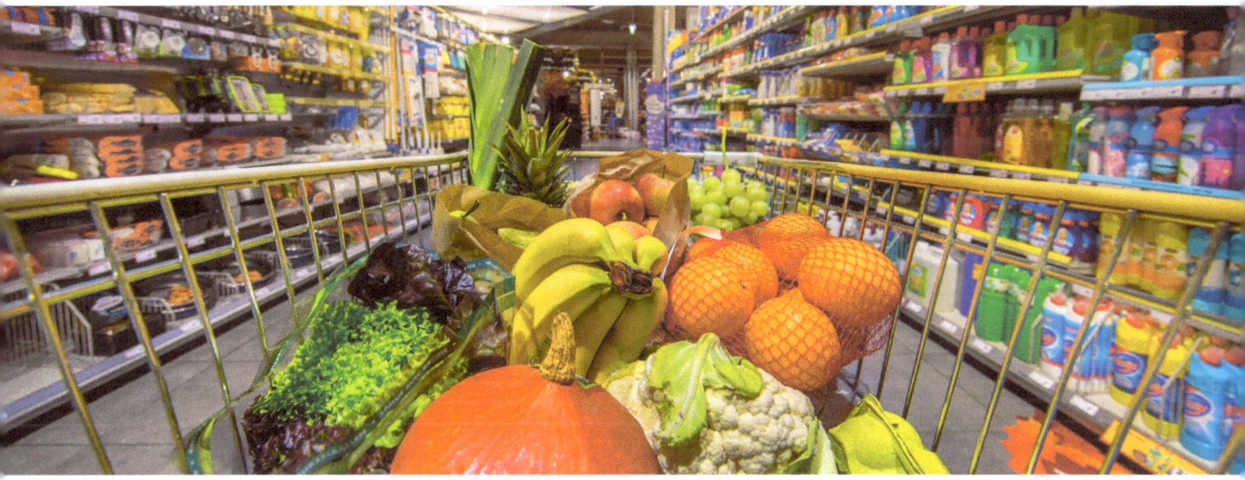

Every meal you eat answers a simple question. Is this food bringing life to my body or slowly draining it of vitality?

Imagine you have two grocery stores on opposite corners of the street. One is filled with "living foods," and the other is filled with "dead" or processed foods. Over the entrance of each store is a giant banner.

One reads: *"Welcome to abundant life. Foods purchased here will give you energy, vitality, clarity of mind, and optimal wellness, while also protecting your body from cancer, strokes, heart attacks, obesity, and other degenerative diseases."*

The other store is worn down but also has a banner with a message in fine print, barely visible to the naked eye.

It reads: *"Our foods taste amazing but are addictive. They are proven to make you more prone to sickness, degenerative diseases, headaches, arthritis, and obesity. While our foods may cause early mortality, you will have fun eating them with your kids, friends, and family. They make the best party snacks and your guests will rave that your place is the funnest place to be!"*

Be honest with yourself, which store do you usually choose? Despite knowing the deadly poisons in foods that are processed, bleached, and with chemicals, most people continue to choose dead foods, hoping they beat the odds.

Before placing something in your cart, ask one simple question. "Is this food supporting life in my body?"

Prioritize Living Foods
Choose foods that come directly from the earth and still carry the life and nutrients God designed them to provide.

Choose Whole Foods
Whenever possible, select foods in their natural form rather than those that have been heavily processed.

Be Mindful of Evening Carbohydrates
As metabolism slows at night, excess carbohydrates are more likely to be stored rather than used for energy. Avoid carbs after 6 pm.

THE LIFE FORCE OF FOOD

God designed food to carry life into our bodies. Fresh fruits, vegetables, nuts, seeds, and naturally raised proteins contain enzymes, vitamins, minerals, and living nutrients that support the body's ability to repair, restore, and produce energy.

But when food is heavily processed, refined, bleached, preserved, or chemically altered, much of that life is lost. What remains may still contain calories, but calories alone do not create vitality. This is why two foods with the same calories can have completely different effects on the body.

Living foods nourish.
Dead foods simply stimulate.

Over time, the body reflects whichever one you choose most often.

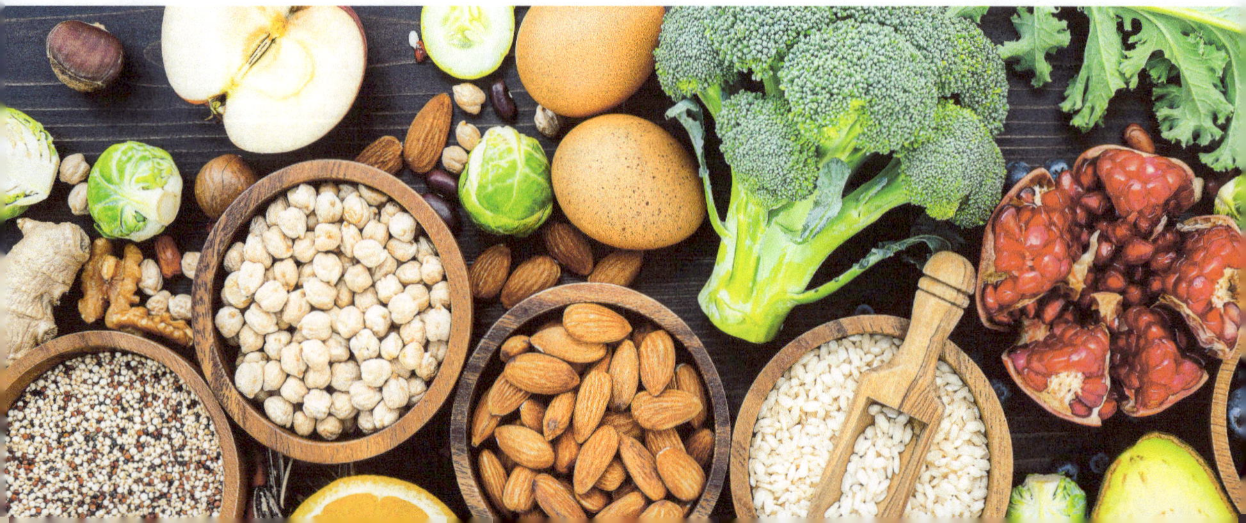

HOW TO READ LABELS

Understanding what is in your food is one of the most powerful steps you can take toward better health. Nutrition labels provide helpful information about calories, fats, carbohydrates, and sodium. Learning to read them helps you make wiser choices and stay aligned with the Fueled plan. Here are a few key terms to understand.

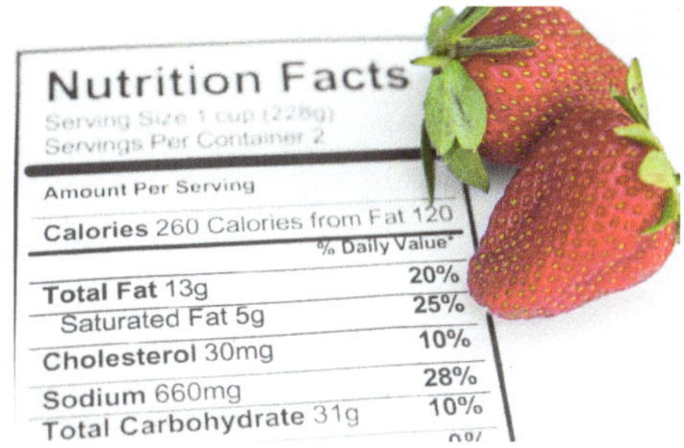
Nutrition Facts
Serving Size 1 cup (228g)
Servings Per Container 2
Amount Per Serving
Calories 260 Calories from Fat 120
% Daily Value*
Total Fat 13g 20%
Saturated Fat 5g 25%
Cholesterol 30mg 10%
Sodium 660mg 28%
Total Carbohydrate 31g 10%

SERVING SIZE

Serving sizes are standardized to make comparisons between similar foods easier. However, they can sometimes be misleading. For example, a pizza box may list 24 grams of fat per serving. That may not sound excessive until you discover that a "serving" might only be one-eighth of a slice. Always check the serving size before evaluating the rest of the label. Knowledge leads to understanding. Understanding leads to wiser decisions.

NOT ALL CALORIES ARE CREATED EQUAL

When it comes to how your body processes food, the quality of calories matters far more than the quantity. Consider two meals that each total 600 calories.

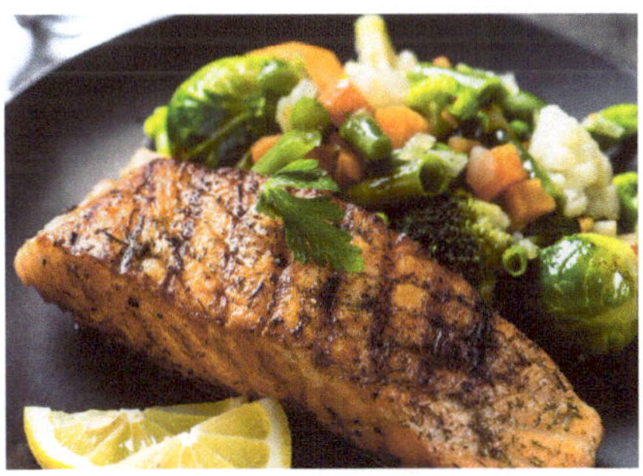

One meal is grilled salmon with vegetables. This meal is rich in fiber, nutrients, and healthy fats. Salmon contains omega-3 fatty acids that support brain health, cardiovascular function, and cellular communication. The protein digests slowly, helping you stay satisfied longer and maintain steady energy.

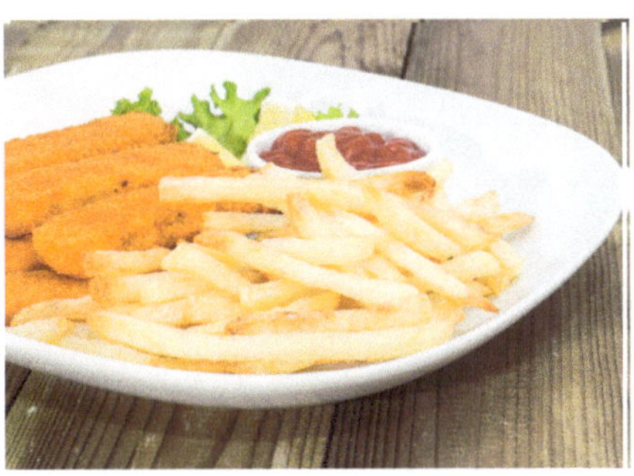

Now compare that to a 600-calorie meal of fish fingers and fries. Despite having the same calorie count, the body processes this meal very differently. Fries are often cooked in inflammatory oils such as canola or sunflower oil and provide little fiber. Ultra-processed fish fingers contain less protein and fewer nutrients than fresh fish. These foods digest quickly, spike blood sugar, and often leave you hungry again shortly afterward. The result is a cycle of energy crashes, cravings, and overeating.

Calories measure the energy in food, but they do not measure the nutritional value that accompanies whole foods. Whole, unprocessed foods provide vitamins, minerals, fiber, and healthy fats that support long-term wellness. Choosing meals like salmon and vegetables instead of highly processed foods is not simply about eating fewer calories. It is about fueling your body with the nutrients it was designed to thrive on.

CHAPTER 7

THE TRUTH ABOUT FATS

God's Design Vs. Man's Distortion

For decades, saturated fats have been demonized and blamed for countless health problems. We were told butter and lard would destroy our hearts, and that the solution was lab-made margarine and highly processed seed oils.

But let's ask the real question. Is that truth, or tradition disguised as science?

Here is a simple Kingdom-minded experiment. Place a stick of butter and a scoop of margarine outside in your backyard. Watch what happens. Ants and animals will gravitate toward the butter, a food that comes from God's creation. Margarine, an artificial imitation made by man, is often left untouched.

Even creation recognizes real food. Butter, lard, and coconut oil are natural foods that have nourished people for generations. Margarine and many industrial seed oils, such as soybean, canola, and sunflower oil, are products of factories, chemical processing, and marketing campaigns. These oils are high in omega-6 fatty acids and can contribute to systemic inflammation when consumed in excess, particularly within the modern Western diet, where the omega-6 to omega-3 ratio is already severely imbalanced.

Over the past several decades, the world embraced the "low-fat" narrative, believing it would lead to longer, healthier lives. The result has been widespread confusion, rising obesity, and increasing rates of chronic illness.

In the past decade alone, major scientific reviews have reexamined the relationship between saturated fat and heart disease. The consistent conclusion is that there is no strong evidence proving saturated fat increases cardiovascular risk.

Yet despite the lack of clear evidence, dietary guidelines still recommend limiting saturated fat to ten percent or less of daily energy intake. Culture often changes more slowly than truth.

A recent analysis of multiple studies found:

- Reducing saturated fat intake likely has little or no effect on overall mortality.
- Evidence that reducing saturated fat lowers coronary heart disease events remains unclear.
- Lowering saturated fat intake appears to have little effect on cardiovascular mortality.

Even LDL cholesterol, the so-called "bad cholesterol," has been widely misunderstood. Research now shows that both extremely low and extremely high LDL levels are associated with increased mortality. An optimal range appears to be around 140 mg/dL (3.6 mmol/L).

In other words, extremes are rarely where health is found. Balance, not fear, should guide our decisions.

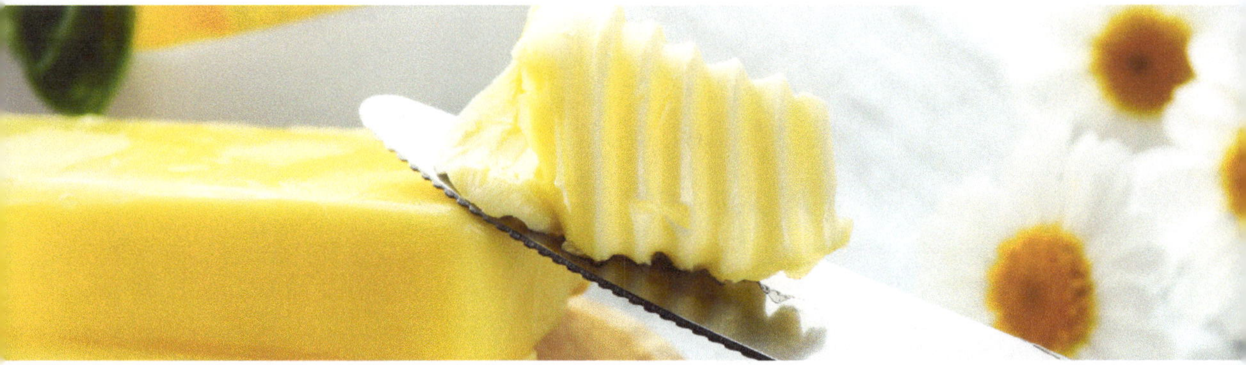

When fat was removed from food, manufacturers had to replace the flavor and texture. The result was an influx of added sugars, starches, and artificial chemicals. What was marketed as "healthy" often became far more harmful.

A "low-fat" yogurt may sound like a good choice until you realize it is packed with sugar, artificial flavorings, and processed thickeners. That is not stewardship of the temple of the Holy Spirit. That is marketing disguised as health.

It is no surprise that metabolic health has declined. God's original design for food still works.

Here is the Kingdom truth. Not all fats are bad. Fake fats are. When we choose foods that are whole, nourishing, and close to the way God created them, we are not only eating better. We are aligning with divine wisdom.

IS FAT OR FAKE FOOD THE REAL VILLIAN?

Let's be honest. Fat never asked for this public relations crisis. Somewhere along the way someone decided fat was responsible for every health problem. Instead of asking, "What kind of fat is this?" the question became, "How quickly can we remove it?"

So food companies stripped fat from everything from yogurt to peanut butter. Then they realized something important. Without fat, food tastes like cardboard. So they went back to the lab and added sugar, artificial flavors, and chemical thickeners to make the food taste good again.

Spoiler alert. Your body is not impressed.

Many so-called "low-fat" foods are now loaded with added sugars, artificial ingredients, and chemical fillers designed to mimic the taste and texture of real food. No wonder so many people feel more tired, inflamed, and confused about what is actually healthy.

Here is the truth.

God is not confused, and neither is your body. When you eat food the way God designed it, full of real, nourishing fats, your body responds. Think avocado, pasture-raised butter, wild-caught salmon, nuts, seeds, and coconut oil. Real food eventually spoils. If something can sit on the counter for weeks without changing, it probably was not real food to begin with.

GOD-MADE FATS VS. FACTORY FATS

A Simple Kitchen Decision Guide

Your brain is nearly 60 percent fat. Your hormones, including estrogen, testosterone, and cortisol, are made from fat. Every cell membrane in your body depends on fat, and vitamins A, D, E, and K require fat for proper absorption.

So when someone says, "I'm cutting all fat to get healthy," what they're really saying is, "I'm starving my brain, confusing my hormones, and blocking my vitamins."

Use this quick guide when stocking your kitchen or shopping at the store.

EAT THESE GOD-MADE FATS	AVOID THESE MAN-MADE FATS
✓ Extra Virgin Olive Oil	✗ Margarine
✓ Avocado Oil	✗ Vegetable Shortening
✓ Coconut Oil	✗ Hydrogenated Oils
✓ Grass-Fed Butter	✗ Soybean Oil
✓ Ghee	✗ Corn Oil
✓ Tallow (Beef Fat)	✗ Grapeseed Oil
✓ Duck Fat	✗ Cottonseed Oil
✓ Avocados	✗ Artificial Butter Substitutes
✓ Nuts & Seeds	✗ Vegetable Oil

SIMPLE RULE

If a fat has to be made in a factory or laboratory, it probably does not belong in your kitchen.

THE QUALITY, QUANTITY, AND FREQUENCY TEST (QQF)

A Kingdom Approach to Discernment in Eating

When it comes to food choices, it is not only what you eat that matters. It is also how much you eat and how often you eat it. That is why we use the QQF Test: Quality, Quantity, and Frequency. This simple framework helps you make wise, Spirit-led decisions that nourish your body, honor your temple, and align with Kingdom stewardship. Before eating, ask yourself three simple questions.

QUALITY

What is the quality of this food? Is it real, whole, and close to the way God created it? Or is it highly processed and manufactured in a factory?

Always choose foods that are organic when possible, minimally processed, and close to their natural state.

QUANTITY

How much of this food am I eating? Even healthy foods should be eaten with wisdom and moderation. A handful of walnuts can support heart health and brain function. But if you are consuming an entire bag every day, your body will store the excess as fat.

Quality matters, but so does balance.

FREQUENCY

How often am I eating this food? Some foods are meant to be daily nourishment. Others should be occasional treats.

For example, a spinach smoothie a few times a week can be beneficial. Drinking two every day for months may lead to excess oxalates, which can contribute to kidney stones. The same principle applies to treats. A slice of cake on a birthday is one thing. A daily habit of sugar-loaded snacks is another story entirely.

When you apply the QQF Test to the food on your plate, you begin to steward your body with intention. Because healthy living is not about rigid rules. It is about wise choices made consistently over time.

How much and what kind of FAT?

Fat is measured in grams. According to the Dietary Guidelines for Americans, adults are encouraged to obtain 20–35 percent of their daily calories from fat. For someone consuming 2,000 calories per day, this typically equals about 45–78 grams of fat. Individual needs may vary depending on health goals and activity levels.

Trans fats are widely recognized as harmful because they contribute to inflammation and increase the risk of heart disease. Margarine is a common example. These highly processed fats can cause cellular damage and should be avoided whenever possible.

Seed and vegetable oils, such as canola, sunflower, and peanut oil, are heavily processed and prone to oxidation when heated. Excess consumption has been linked to inflammation and metabolic stress within the body.

Monounsaturated fats, such as olive oil, are considered beneficial fats. Extra virgin olive oil contains antioxidants and anti-inflammatory compounds that support heart health. Use it regularly but in moderation, as all fats are calorie-dense.

Saturated fats such as pasture-raised butter, ghee, lard, tallow, duck fat, coconut oil, and eggs have nourished cultures for generations. These fats tend to be more stable at higher temperatures, making them suitable for cooking. As with all foods, balance and moderation remain important.

CARBOHYDRATES

Carbohydrates provide energy for the body, supporting everything from daily movement to intense physical activity. Whenever possible, choose carbohydrates that come from whole, natural sources such as vegetables, fruits, and other plant-based foods rather than refined carbohydrates like white bread and processed snacks. Because the body's metabolism naturally slows in the evening, limit carbohydrate intake after 6:00 p.m.

PROTEIN

Protein supports the body's ability to build and repair tissues, maintain muscle mass, and sustain metabolic function. The average American diet includes protein from meat, poultry, fish, eggs, and other animal sources, though beans, nuts, and seeds also provide valuable protein. Quality matters. Grass-fed meats and wild-caught fish tend to provide higher nutrient density while reducing exposure to added hormones, antibiotics, pesticides, and other chemical inputs.

Food is more than fuel for the stomach. It is fuel for every cell in your body. The nutrents you choose each day determine how well your cells produce energy, repair damage, and sustain life. In the next chapter, we will explore the tiny power plants inside your cells that make this possible. They are called **mitochondria.**

WEEKLY FOOD TRACKER

On a separate piece of paper or on the back of this one, keep a log of EVERYTHING you eat, drink, suck on, or chew. This will be important if you want to discover your blind spots or areas of nutritional weakness that might be sabotaging your results in other areas of life.

	Sunday	Monday	Tuesday	Wednesday	Thursday	Friday	Saturday
How much water did you drink?							
How many hours did you sleep?							
What was your stress level (0 -5)							
What did you do for physical exercise?							
On average, did you eat more living or dead foods?							
What was the first thing you ate or drank today and when?							
What did you eat for breakfast and at what time?							
Today's snacks: candy, gum, etc. and at what time?							
Lunch							
Dinner							

Did you eat anything after 6 p.m.? If so, what was it and at what time? ______________________

CHAPTER 8

MITOCHONDRIA

The Powerhouse of Your Cells

Energy is the currency of life.

Just like money in the bank, it's exciting to spend, difficult to earn, and dangerous to run out of. When your energy account is full, life feels vibrant. Your mind is clear. Your body moves with strength. Your purpose feels within reach.

But when that account runs low, everything becomes harder. Focus fades. Motivation disappears. Even simple tasks feel exhausting. Inside every one of your cells are tiny structures responsible for managing this energy economy. They are called "mitochondria," and they function as the power plants of your body. Their job is simple but extraordinary: they convert the food you eat and the oxygen you breathe into ATP, the biological energy that fuels every heartbeat, every thought, and every movement.

But here's the truth: Fatigue isn't just exhaustion; it's a warning light on your life's dashboard. You can't run on empty and expect peak performance.

Think of your body like a high-performance Formula 1 race car. An F1 car is engineered for speed, endurance, and precision. But even the best car on the track will fail without three things:

- high-quality fuel
- efficient oxygen flow
- a finely tuned engine

Your body works the same way. Your mitochondria are the engine. Your lungs supply oxygen. Your digestive system provides the fuel. And when these systems work together, energy flows effortlessly.

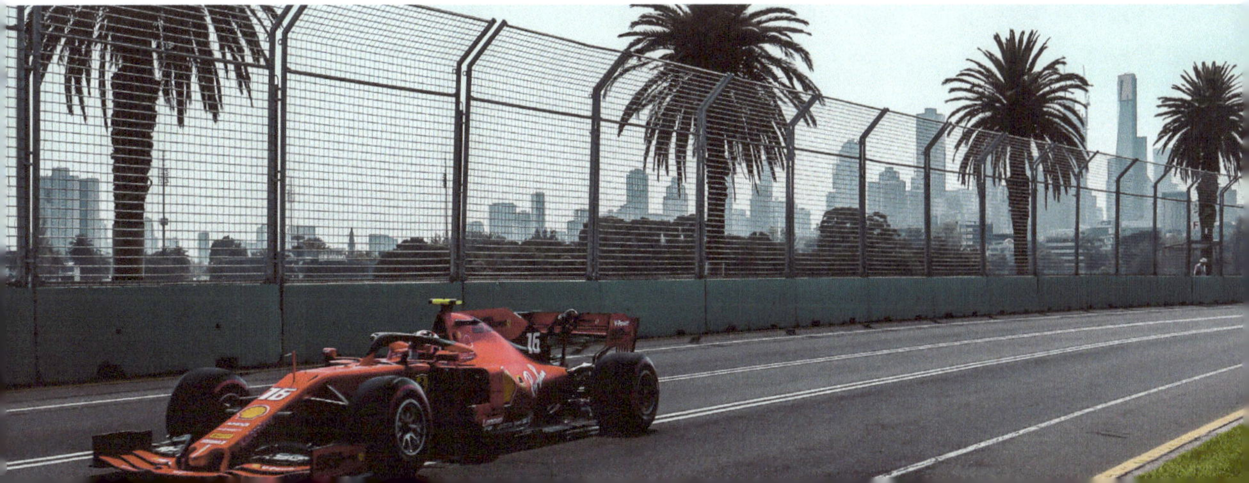

This table highlights the synergy between maintaining an F1 car's performance and ensuring optimal human health through mitochondrial care. Both require precise management, maintenance, and high-quality inputs for peak performance.

F1 Car Component	Role in the F1 Car	Human Body Equivalent	Role in the Body
Engine	Powers the car	**Mitochondria**	Produces energy (ATP) for the body
Fuel	High-performance fuel	**Nutrition & Gut Function**	Provides essential nutrients for energy
Oxygen Intake	Air intake system	**Lungs**	Delivers oxygen to the bloodstream
Fuel & Oxygen Delivery	Fuel injection system	**Heart & Circulation**	Transports fuel (nutrients) and oxygen
Accelerator Pedal	Controls speed and performance	**Thyroid**	Regulates metabolism and energy output
Gearbox	Adjusts speed and power distribution	**Adrenal Glands**	Manages stress response and energy flow
Service & Repair	Regular maintenance and pit stops	**Sleep**	Restores and repairs body functions
Tool Kit	Essential maintenance tools	**Methylation Cycle**	Supports detoxification and cell repair
Cleaning Oil	Lubricates engine, prevents breakdown	**Antioxidants**	Protects cells from oxidative damage
Catalytic Converter	Reduces harmful emissions	**Detoxification System**	Eliminates toxins from the body
Driver	Skilled operator for optimal performance	**Brain (Fit & Focused)**	Directs decisions and body coordination

The average cell uses an astonishing ten billion ATP molecules per day! Since ATP can't be stored, our bodies must produce their entire weight in ATP daily to sustain essential functions like hormone production, toxin elimination, and muscle contraction, including the beating of our hearts.

About two-thirds of our energy goes toward simply staying alive (known as the basal metabolic rate, or BMR), while the remaining third fuels our physical and mental activities. Given this critical role, it's vital to care for the incredible, God-designed powerhouses within us, our mitochondria. These tiny structures fuel the energy, vitality, and endurance we need to fulfill our Kingdom purpose and live out our God-given potential.

GOD'S TINY POWER PLANTS

Every engine produces exhaust. As your mitochondria generate energy, they also produce small by-products called "free radicals." These molecules are unstable and reactive. In scientific terms, they are known as "reactive oxygen species, or ROS."

Think of them like microscopic sparks flying off an engine. In small amounts, they are normal. In fact, they even play useful roles in signaling within the body.

But when too many accumulate, those sparks start causing damage. Cells begin to rust from the inside out. This process, called oxidative stress, is linked to fatigue, inflammation, accelerated aging, and many chronic diseases.

But here's the good news: God designed your body with an incredible defense system. Built directly into your cells is a network of antioxidants that neutralize these harmful by-products and keep your cellular engines running smoothly.

Think of them as your body's built-in maintenance crew, constantly cleaning up the microscopic exhaust produced by energy generation. When your antioxidant defenses are strong, your cells stay resilient.

The First Warning Light: Fatigue

Just like a car's check engine light signals a problem under the hood, your body sends signals too. If you're constantly tired, mentally foggy, and feeling like your "get-up-and-go" got up and went... chances are, your mitochondria are waving a little white flag.

And here's an amazing fact: A healthy body generates around 1,200 watts of energy every single day, and around 70 percent of that energy is used by your brain!

Your energy isn't just for workouts or chasing toddlers. It powers your thoughts, focus, emotions, and spiritual stamina. When your mitochondria are thriving, so are you.

So What Damages These Mighty Mitochondria? Here are a few of the top culprits that can sabotage your cellular power plants:

- Oxidative stress from a poor diet or chronic inflammation.
- Aging (natural, but can be slowed with good stewardship).
- Toxic metals and industrial chemicals (hello, pesticides and pollution).
- Alcohol (sorry, but your mitochondria aren't toasting with you).
- Overuse of certain medications, such as:
  - Acetaminophen
  - Aspirin
  - Antibiotics
  - Statins
  - NSAIDs (like ibuprofen)

MITOCHONDRIA... THE UNSUNG HEROS OF HEALTH

Your mitochondria were designed to sustain your life force, your calling, and your Kingdom assignment. They work quietly behind the scenes every second of every day, generating the energy that allows your heart to beat, your brain to think, and your body to move. You may never see them, but their impact touches every part of your health. In many ways, mitochondria are the unsung heroes of human vitality.

Here are just a few of their lesser-known, but incredibly important roles:

Nutrient Metabolism
Mitochondria help break down and convert nutrients into usable energy, supporting thousands of biological processes necessary for optimal health.

Aging
Mitochondrial dysfunction is closely linked to the aging process. In fact, one reason fasting is associated with longevity is that it boosts mitochondrial function by increasing the NAD+/NADH ratio, a key marker of cellular vitality.

Lipid Metabolism
Did you know? The mitochondria help regulate fat metabolism, including the production of cholesterol and other lipids essential for hormone synthesis and cellular health.

Drug & Toxin Detoxification
They also play a role in detoxifying medications and environmental chemicals—working like the body's internal hazmat crew.

Stress Hormone Production
Your mitochondria help produce cortisol and other hormones that manage the stress response. If they're not working well, you may find yourself burning out faster than you can pray it away.

Growth & Repair (Especially Gut Health!)
The cells lining your gut wall regenerate rapidly, and guess who helps fuel that constant renewal? You got it: your mitochondria.

Healthy mitochondria = stronger gut = better immunity and nutrient absorption.

Glucose & Insulin Regulation
They help regulate blood sugar and insulin sensitivity, which impacts heart health, metabolism, weight, and risk for type 2 diabetes. Dysfunction here is a major driver of metabolic syndrome.

Hormone Signaling
Mitochondria help coordinate hormone signaling throughout the body. When impaired, this can contribute to hormonal imbalances, reproductive challenges, and irregular cycles.

Brain & Nervous System Function
Your brain is one of the most energy-hungry organs in your body and when your mitochondria aren't functioning well, you'll feel it. Brain fog, trouble concentrating, memory lapses, mood swings, anxiety, depression, and even neurological diseases like Alzheimer's and Parkinson's can all be linked to mitochondrial dysfunction.

Immune System Function
Mitochondria produce reactive oxygen species (ROS) that help regulate immune responses. When this process is off balance, it can contribute to immune system breakdown, increasing your risk for infections, inflammation, and even autoimmunity.

Your mitochondria are doing way more than just keeping the lights on. They're deeply involved in how you think, feel, move, heal, and age. If you want to live with energy, clarity, and long-term vitality—it's time to bless your mitochondria with the nutrition, movement, rest, and spiritual alignment they need. Because when these little powerhouses are Fueled properly... so are you.

FUELING YOUR MITOCHONDRIA

Like any engine, mitochondria require specific nutrients to function efficiently. These nutrients support energy production, protect cells from damage, and help maintain metabolic balance.

When you fuel your mitochondria with nutrient-dense foods, hydration, oxygen, and rest, they keep you energized, sharp, and resilient. But when you feed them processed junk, live in chronic stress, or neglect sleep, your energy tanks, your hormones misfire, and your metabolism slows to a crawl. In Kingdom terms? When your internal temple isn't fueled properly, your assignment becomes harder to carry out. Healthy mitochondria = sustainable Kingdom impact.

What mitochondria need to thrive:
- Food (nutrients)
- Oxygen(movement and exercise)

And three key micronutrients:
- Copper
- Magnesium
- B Vitamins

Other powerful nutrients that support mitochondrial health include:
CoQ10, Alpha-Lipoic Acid, Acetyl-L-Carnitine, Resveratrol, NAC (N-Acetyl-Cysteine), and Vitamin E.

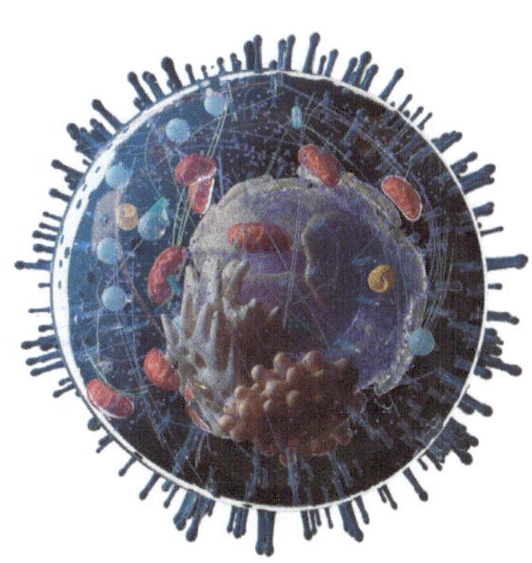

6 WAYS TO FUEL YOUR MITOCHONDRIA

Eat to Fuel Your Cells

Food is your fuel! The better the quality, the better your "engine" runs. Prioritize real, nutrient-dense foods to reduce oxidative stress and boost energy.

Limit Toxin Exposure

Toxins are everywhere. They are in food, products, and even furniture. Reduce what goes in, and support your body's ability to clear what's already there. (See more tips in the "Hormonal Health" chapter.)

Build Muscle with Exercise

Movement, especially strength training and HIIT (high-intensity interval training), boosts mitochondrial growth. More muscle = more mitochondria = more energy!

Avoid Overeating

Calorie overload creates inflammation and oxidative stress. Strategic fasting or mindful eating helps your mitochondria multiply and function better.

Manage Stress

Chronic stress drains the nutrients your mitochondria need to thrive. Build rhythms of rest and trust God's peace to recharge your body and mind.

Get Deep, Restorative Sleep

Sleep is when your body repairs and resets. Poor sleep disrupts mitochondrial health and throws your hormones off balance. Prioritize your bedtime like your health depends on it, because it does.

When you care for your mitochondria, you're not just boosting energy; you're honoring the temple God gave you. And when your cellular engines are Fueled well, your life begins to reflect it. Your mind becomes sharper. Your body grows stronger. Your calling becomes easier to carry.

"Do you not know that your bodies are temples of the Holy Spirit, who is in you, whom you have received from God? You are not your own; you were bought at a price. Therefore, honor God with your bodies."
— 1 Corinthians 6:19-20

THE ENERGY EQUATION

Energy Production = Nutrition + Oxygen + Movement + Rest

When these work together, the body produces the vitality you were designed to experience.

CHAPTER 9
YOUR GUT GARDEN

Where Your Health Begins to Grow

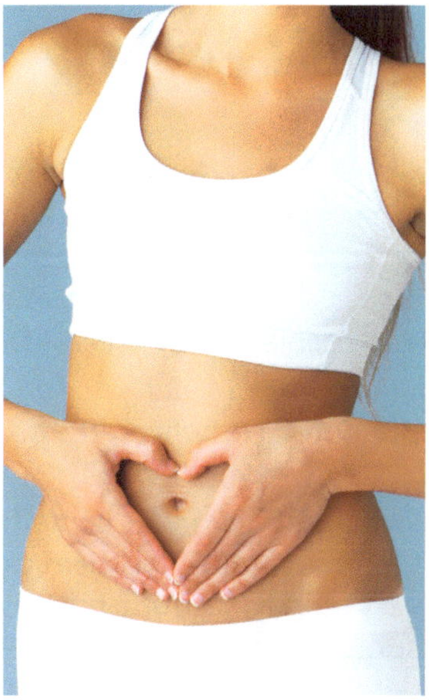

Imagine your gut as a living garden. In this garden, trillions of tiny organisms work together to keep the soil healthy and productive. Just like the insects and earthworms that help plants grow, beneficial bacteria in your gut nurture the internal environment that sustains your health.

In this internal garden, beneficial bacteria act like the diligent workers of the soil. They strengthen immune defenses, produce essential vitamins, and help break down the complex foods we eat. They also help regulate weight and protect us from harmful invaders such as Candida and other pathogens.

Your gut also constantly communicates with the rest of your body through powerful signaling networks known as the "gut-brain," "gut-skin," "gut-hormone," and "gut-thyroid" axes. You've probably experienced this connection firsthand. When you're nervous before a big presentation or stressful event, it's often your gut that reacts first.

More than 90% of the body's serotonin—the neurotransmitter linked to mood and well-being is produced in the gut. When gut bacteria fall out of balance, the effects can ripple throughout the body, influencing everything from mood and anxiety to skin health and immune function.

When gut bacteria become imbalanced, people are more vulnerable to a wide range of issues including brain fog, anxiety, depression, mood disorders, and skin conditions such as eczema and psoriasis.

Think of it this way: if a garden becomes overrun with weeds and lacks the insects that help maintain the soil, the entire ecosystem struggles. In the same way, when harmful microbes crowd out beneficial ones, the gut enters a state known as "dysbiosis," and health begins to decline.

> *You are not just feeding yourself. You are feeding the trillions of microbes that help determine your health.*

THE GLUCOSE ROLLER COASTER

Have you ever noticed how some days you feel unstoppable, while other days even small tasks feel exhausting? One moment your energy is high, your focus is sharp, and you feel motivated and clear-headed. A few hours later, you are tired, irritable, and reaching for another cup of coffee or something sweet just to make it through the afternoon.

That isn't a lack of discipline.

It's biology.

When you eat a meal high in carbohydrates, those carbohydrates are broken down into glucose. This glucose enters your bloodstream, prompting your pancreas to release insulin. Insulin helps move glucose into your cells, where your mitochondria convert it into usable energy called ATP. This is how the body was designed to create energy.

But not all carbohydrates behave the same way.

When carbohydrates come from processed or ultra-processed foods, they can send your blood sugar on a biochemical roller coaster. Foods that are stripped of fiber are digested very quickly, causing blood sugar to spike rapidly. In response, your pancreas releases a surge of insulin to bring those levels down. Sometimes it brings them down too far.

This sudden drop in blood sugar, known as "hypoglycemia," can leave you feeling exhausted, foggy, irritable, and craving quick sources of energy like sugar or caffeine to bring your levels back up again.

And just like that, the cycle repeats.

Up.
Down.
Spike.
Crash.

Over time, this constant metabolic roller coaster places tremendous stress on the body and can contribute to long-term health issues such as insulin resistance, obesity, type 2 diabetes, and cardiovascular disease.

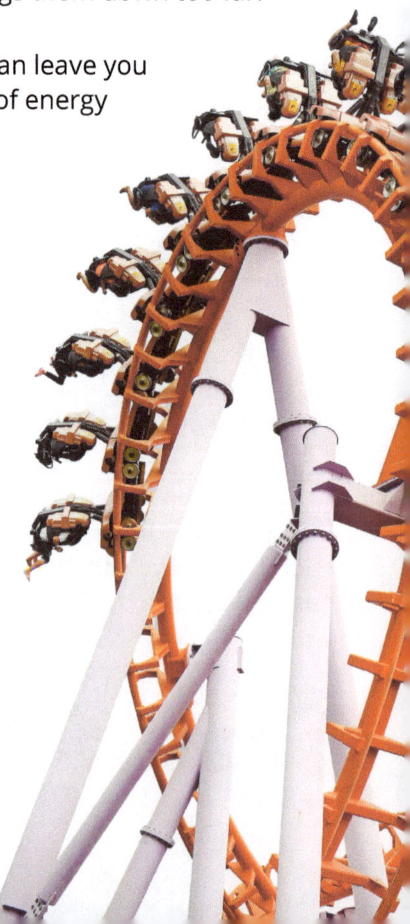

The good news is that stabilizing this roller coaster is surprisingly simple. When you choose whole, fiber-rich foods, digestion slows down. Glucose enters the bloodstream more gradually, allowing insulin to respond in a steady and balanced way.

Instead of dramatic spikes and crashes, foods like vegetables, whole grains, and legumes provide complex carbohydrates that nourish your body while supporting stable blood sugar levels. The result is sustained energy, clearer thinking, and a body that functions as it was designed to. A steady body supports a steady life, giving you the strength to live out the purpose God designed you for.

The solution begins with what you place on your plate.

ARE YOU ON A BLOOD SUGAR ROLLER COASTER?

- You feel energized after eating, but crash within a few hours.
- You rely on caffeine just to get through the afternoon.
- You feel shaky, irritable, or anxious when meals are delayed.
- You crave sugar or quick carbohydrates between meals.
- Your mood swings throughout the day.
- You experience brain fog or trouble concentrating.
- You feel hungry again shortly after eating.
- Your energy improves briefly after sweets, then drops again.

The encouraging news is that this cycle can often be corrected by stabilizing your meals with fiber-rich foods, healthy fats, and quality protein, slowing digestion and supporting steady energy.

Strategies for A HAPPY GUT

Remember the garden analogy. Just as a garden can suffer from poor soil, harsh chemicals, pests, and lack of sunlight, your gut can be affected by low stomach acid, medications, infections, poor diet, stress, excessive cleanliness, urban environments, and C-section births.

The encouraging news is that, like a garden, your gut can thrive with the right care. When you nourish the soil, support beneficial microbes, and provide the nutrients they need, your internal ecosystem becomes stronger and more resilient.

With the right nutrition and lifestyle habits, your gut can flourish.

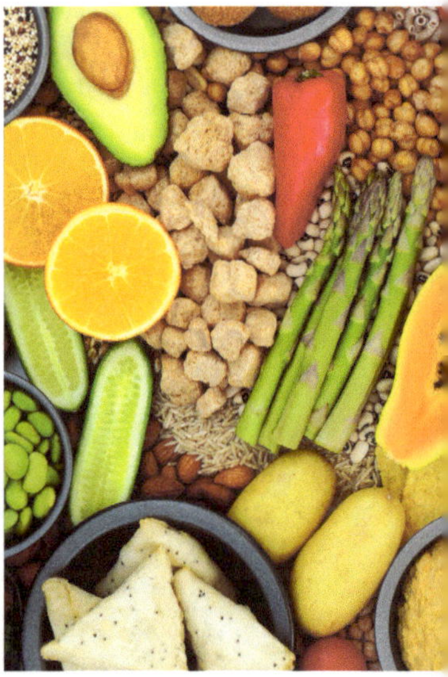

PLANT FOOD DIVERSITY

More Fiber, More Polyphenols, and Better Nutrients

Increasing the variety of plant foods in your diet is one of the most powerful ways to improve gut health. When you aim to eat thirty-five different plant foods each week, you help strengthen the diversity of beneficial bacteria in your gut. Plant foods include fruits, vegetables, beans, whole grains, nuts, seeds, herbs, and spices. Even different colors of the same food count separately. For example, red, yellow, and green bell peppers each contain unique plant compounds called "polyphenols" that nourish gut bacteria. This means reaching thirty-five plant foods each week is more achievable than it sounds.

TIP: Try introducing one new fruit, vegetable, herb, spice, or nut each week. If you enjoy it, add it to your regular meals. If not, try something new the following week. Over the course of a year, even adding fifty new plant foods to your diet can dramatically increase the diversity of nutrients that support your gut and overall health.

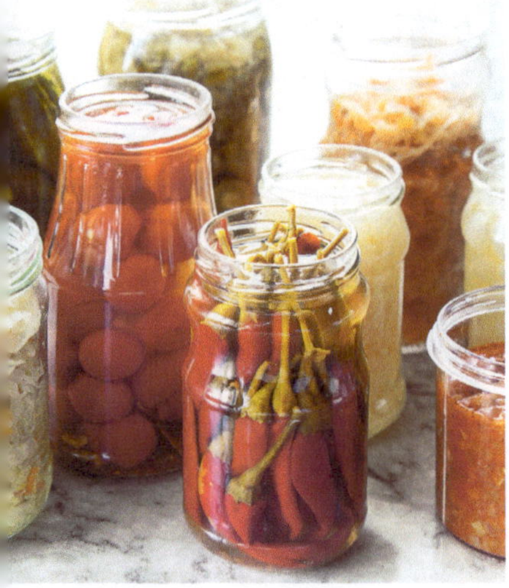

FERMENTED FOODS

Fermented foods are another powerful way to strengthen your gut microbiome. These foods contain beneficial bacteria that support digestion, strengthen immunity, and help maintain a balanced gut environment. Unlike many probiotic supplements, fermented foods naturally deliver a wide range of living microbes. Examples include sauerkraut, fermented vegetables, apple cider vinegar, kimchi, tempeh, miso, yogurt, kefir, and certain fermented cheeses. Regularly including these foods in your diet can help support a healthy balance of beneficial bacteria.

A thriving gut creates a thriving body and a thriving life.

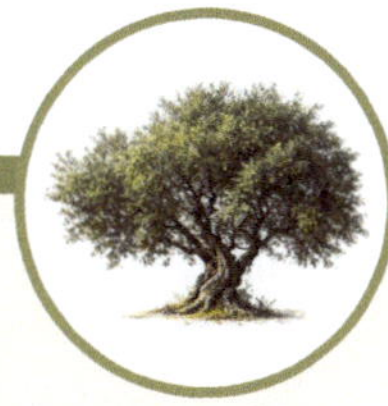

GUT GARDEN CHECKLIST

SIMPLE HABITS THAT HELP YOUR MICROBIOME THRIVE

☐ I eat a variety of plant foods each week, including fruits, vegetables, beans, nuts, seeds, herbs, and spices.

☐ I aim to consume about thirty-five different plant foods during the week.

☐ I include fiber-rich foods such as leafy greens, legumes, and whole grains.

☐ I regularly eat fermented foods such as yogurt, kefir, sauerkraut, kimchi, or fermented vegetables.

☐ I limit highly processed foods that can disrupt beneficial bacteria.

☐ I drink enough water to support digestion and nutrient absorption.

☐ I manage stress through prayer, rest, movement, or time outdoors.

☐ I avoid unnecessary antibiotics and medications when possible.

☐ I spend time outdoors, where exposure to natural microbes can support microbial diversity.

☐ I choose whole foods that nourish my body rather than ultra-processed foods that weaken gut health.

"The Lord God took the man and put him in the Garden of Eden to work it and take care of it."

— Genesis 2:15

CHAPTER 10

THE BALANCED PLATE

Fueling Your Body the Way God Designed

For many people, nutrition can feel confusing. New diets pop up every year. One expert says avoid carbs, and another says avoid fats. Labels are complicated, and meal planning can feel overwhelming.

But nourishing your body does not have to be complicated. When you turn to whole foods and build meals with the right balance of nutrients, your body naturally begins to stabilize energy, support digestion, and reduce cravings.

Instead of dramatic spikes and crashes, your body receives a steady stream of nourishment that fuels your cells and supports long-term health.

One of the easiest ways to do this is by using a simple visual guide called **The Balanced Plate.** Think of every meal as an opportunity to fuel your body well and steward it with wise choices.

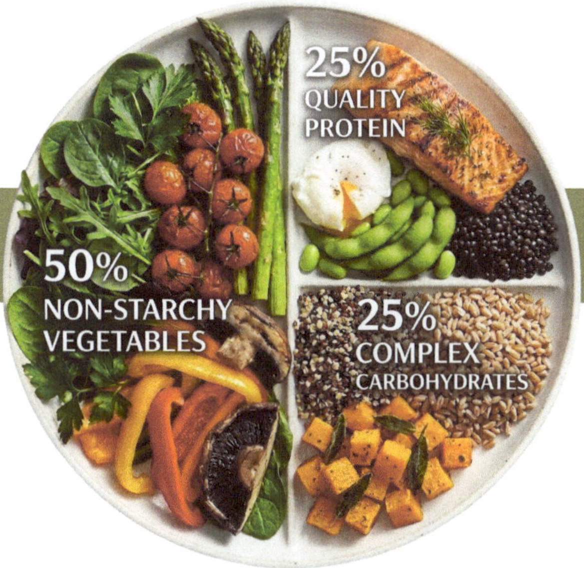

50% of your plate = non-starchy vegetables

25% of your plate = quality protein

25% of your plate = complex carbohydrates

- **50% Non-Starchy Vegetables**
  - Fill half your plate with high-fiber vegetables that grow above the ground. These are vegetables that are rich in fiber, vitamins, minerals, and plant compounds that nourish your gut bacteria and support stable blood sugar levels.
  - Leafy greens, broccoli, cauliflower, peppers, zucchini, cabbage, cucumbers, mushrooms, and asparagus are all excellent choices. When half your plate is filled with vegetables, your body receives the nutrients it needs to function well.
- **25% High-Quality Protein**
  - Protein supports muscle repair, immune health, hormone balance, and steady energy. It also slows digestion and helps prevent blood sugar spikes.
  - Healthy protein choices include wild-caught fish, grass-fed meats, eggs, poultry, beans, lentils, tofu, and tempeh. Including protein at every meal also helps you feel satisfied longer.
- **25% Complex Carbohydrates:**
  - Carbohydrates are not the enemy. Your body uses them as a source of fuel. The key is choosing carbohydrates that come from whole foods rather than highly processed products.
  - Complex carbohydrates such as sweet potatoes, quinoa, brown rice, beans, lentils, and whole grains provide fiber and nutrients that support steady energy levels.These foods digest more slowly and help avoid the glucose spikes that lead to fatigue and cravings.

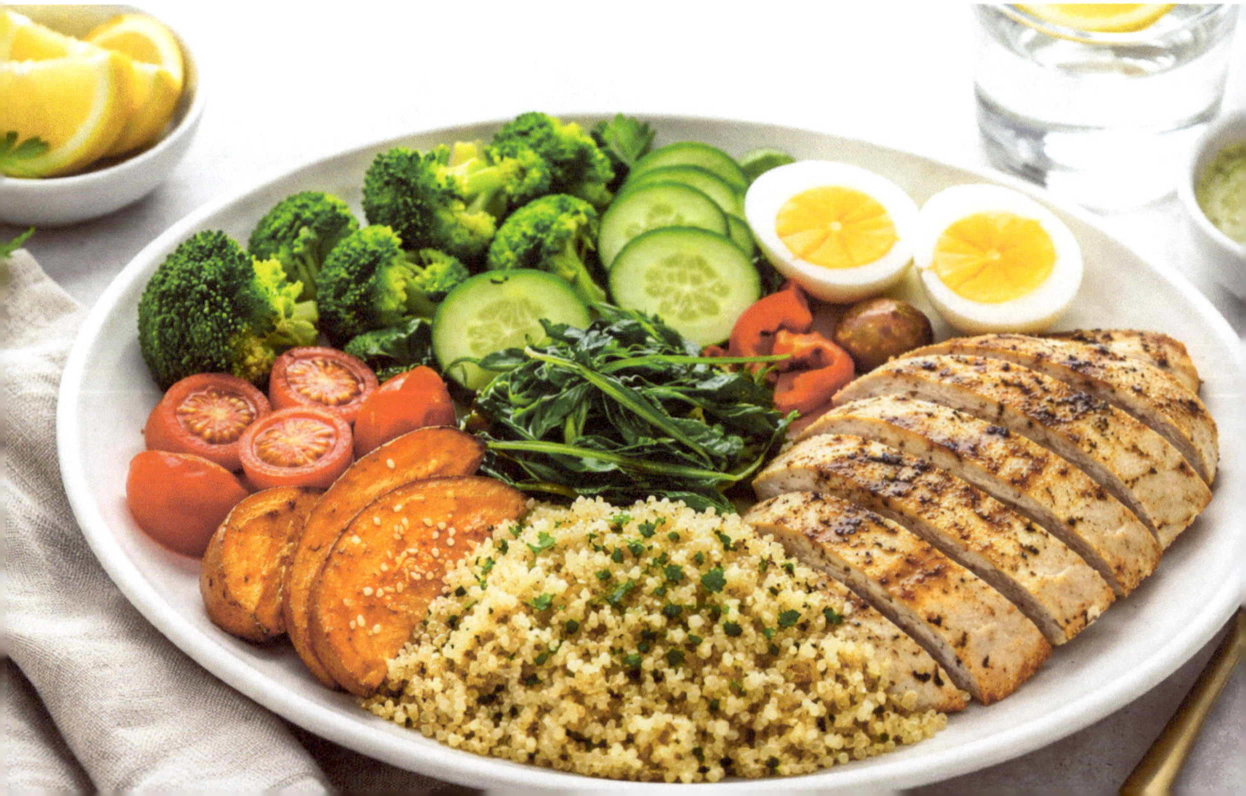

EATING WITH PURPOSE NOT DISTRACTION

Eating at your desk, in front of the television, or while scrolling through your phone may feel efficient, but it often comes at a cost.

When we eat distracted, we stop paying attention to our body's signals. The same plate of food can nourish you very differently depending on whether you eat it mindfully or while multitasking.

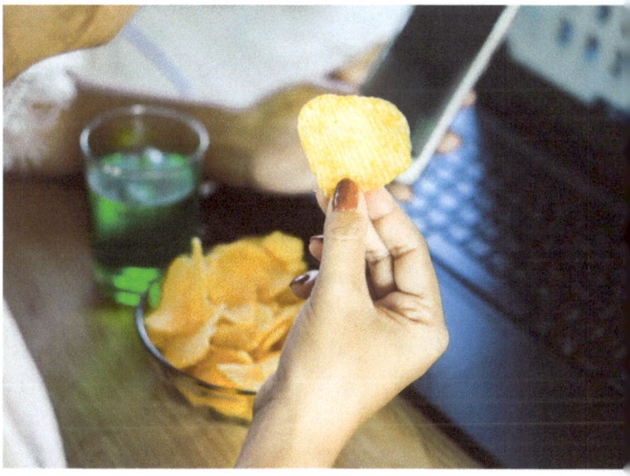

In today's fast-paced world, mindless eating has quietly become the norm. We grab lunch on the go, snack for a quick energy boost, and unwind at night with dinner in front of a screen. In the process, we lose awareness of what we are eating and why.

Have you ever opened the refrigerator, stood there staring for a moment, and reached for something even though you were not truly hungry?

You are not alone.

Researchers have identified several common eating patterns driven by habit or emotion rather than genuine hunger. According to Dr. Helen McCarthy, The Appetite Doctor, there are five common forms of non-hunger eating.

Habitual Eating - Eating simply because it is a certain time of day or part of a routine.

Opportunistic Eating - Grabbing food because it is available or placed in front of you.

Insurance Policy Eating - Eating "just in case" you might get hungry later.

Craving-Based Eating - Responding to desires rather than true physical hunger.

Emotional Eating - Using food to cope with stress, boredom, or uncomfortable emotions.

Over time, these patterns can lead to weight gain, blood sugar imbalance, and long-term health challenges. At the center of all of them is the same issue.

Mindless eating.

Ask yourself a simple question before eating.
Am I truly hungry, or am I simply responding to habit, emotion, or convenience?

THE POWER OF MINDFUL EATING

The cephalic phase is a remarkable process that is triggered by your senses. The sight of a beautiful meal, the aroma rising from the plate, or the sizzle of food cooking signals your brain that nourishment is on the way.

Your body immediately begins preparing. In response, your God-designed digestive system activates.

- Saliva releases enzymes that begin breaking down carbohydrates in your mouth.
- Your stomach begins producing acid to digest protein.
- Your pancreas releases enzymes that help convert food into usable nutrients.
- Your gallbladder sends bile to help digest fats.

But here's the problem.

This remarkable digestive sequence works best when you are fully present. If you are eating at your desk, scrolling through your phone, or watching television, your brain never fully registers that food has arrived. Your body does not respond the way it was designed to.

This is called "mindless eating," and over time, it can lead to poor digestion, bloating, missed nutrient absorption, and a constant feeling of dissatisfaction after meals.

So what does MINDFUL eating look like?

It begins with something very simple.

Presence.

Mindful eating means slowing down, giving thanks, and engaging intentionally with the senses that God has given you.

- Look at your food. Notice the colors and presentation.
- Smell the aroma. Let your senses prepare your body for nourishment.
- Taste each bite. Slow down and enjoy it.
- Chew intentionally. Digestion begins in the mouth.
- Remove distractions. Your body can't digest what your brain doesn't acknowledge.

This is so much more than a nutritional habit. Mindful eating is a spiritual discipline. When you slow down and eat with intention, you honor the food God has provided, and you honor the body He's entrusted to you.

The next time you sit down for a meal, resist the urge to multitask. Instead, pause, give thanks, engage your senses, and enjoy!

7 WAYS TO IMPROVE DIGESTION AND EAT MORE MINDFULLY

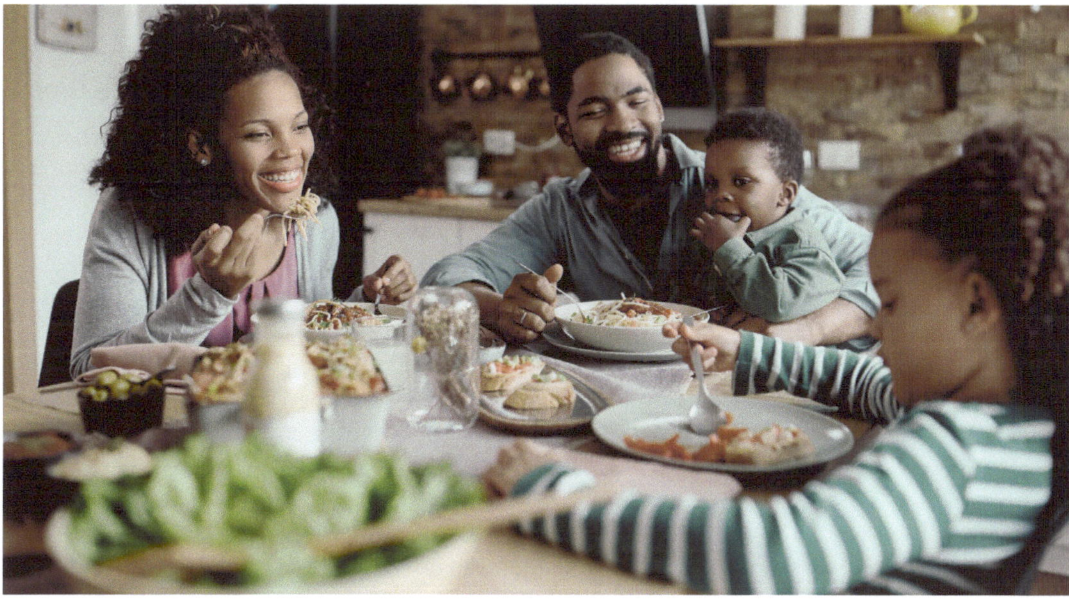

Digestion begins long before the first bite reaches your stomach.

The way you prepare your food, the pace of your meal, and even the atmosphere around the table all influence how well your body receives nourishment.

These small habits help your body shift into the state it was designed for: rest, digest, and restore.

Cook Your Food or Warm It on the Stove

Engaging your senses while cooking helps activate digestion before your first bite. If you cannot cook from scratch, warming food gently on the stove rather than in the microwave can still help create a slower, more intentional start to the meal.

Eat at the Table, Not at Your Desk

Your environment sends powerful signals to your body. Sitting at a table creates a designated space for nourishment and helps your brain shift out of work mode and into mealtime.

Slow Down & Chew Thoroughly

Chewing is one of the simplest and most effective ways to support digestion. Aim for twenty to thirty chews per bite. This allows enzymes in your saliva to begin breaking down food before it reaches your stomach.

Put Away Devices While Eating

Scrolling your phone, answering emails, or watching television keeps your brain distracted. When your brain does not fully register a meal, digestion and fullness signals become less effective.

Breathe Deeply Before You Eat

Take two minutes for slow breathing before beginning your meal. Inhale for four seconds, hold for four seconds, exhale for four seconds, and pause for four seconds. This shifts your body from a stress response into a relaxed digestive state.

Don't Eat When You're Stressed

If you're in the middle of a high-stress moment and can't calm down first, it's better to delay your meal. Eating while tense shuts down digestion and can cause discomfort.

Share Meals with Loved Ones When Possible

Eating with family or friends encourages slower, more mindful eating and naturally lowers stress levels. The emotional connection enhances the physical nourishment.

When you slow down and honor the process of eating, nourishment becomes more than a biological act. It becomes an act of stewardship for the body God entrusted to you.

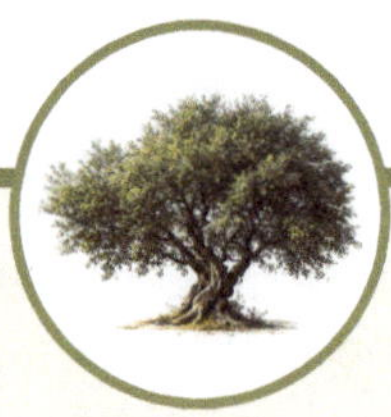

DIGESTION BEGINS WITH PEACE

Your body digests best in a calm state.

Rushing, multitasking, and stressing interrupt this process.

Slow down... Give thanks...

Let your body receive nourishment the way it was designed.

In Peace.

FOOD DIVERSITY TRACKER

Track the variety of plant foods you eat below, including fruits, vegetables, seeds, nuts, herbs, and spices. Count different colors or types separately (e.g., green, yellow, and red bell peppers each count as one). Each plant food counts only once per week, no matter how often you eat it.

	Sunday	Monday	Tuesday	Wednesday	Thursday	Friday	Saturday
Plant food 1							
Plant food 2							
Plant food 3							
Plant food 4							
Plant food 5							
Plant food 6							
Plant food 7							
Plant food 8							
Plant food 9							
Total plant foods consumed per day							

Total plant foods consumed this week: ______________________

CHAPTER 11

HORMONAL HARMONY

Your Body–God's Symphony

There is a moment in every person's life when their body quietly whispers:

Something has changed.

For me, that moment happened in the passenger seat of Larry's truck while I was cycling through four climate zones in ten minutes.

I had joyfully entered perimenopause at forty-eight. And once again, I made a firm decision.

I was not going to be one of those women.

You know the ones I'm talking about.

Hot flashes.
Mood swings.
Emotional hijackings.

I was convinced my healthy lifestyle and spiritual discipline had somehow earned me a lifetime exemption.

Then my fifties arrived.

And suddenly Larry's truck thermostat started living its own life.

A/C up.
A/C down.
Heater on.
Heater off.
Windows open.
Windows closed.
Shirt off...

Just kidding. I kept my clothes on.

But bless Larry's heart. He rode through more climate zones in that truck than a Delta flight from Dallas to Iceland.

One day, he looked over at me cautiously. The way a man approaches a sleeping bear.

"Honey… do you think you might be having hot flashes?"

Let's just say those were fighting words.

The truth is, no matter how disciplined we try to be, there are moments in life when life simply happens. Not because God has abandoned us. Sometimes it is because He is teaching us something we could only learn through experience.

That season taught me something humbling. Never judge someone for a struggle you believe could never happen to you.

Jesus warned about this very thing in Matthew 7:

"Do not judge, or you too will be judged… with the measure you use, it will be measured to you."

Now, when I see someone wrestling with something I once thought I would never face, I don't judge them.

I pray for them.

Because life has a way of reminding us that when we point one finger at someone else, three fingers are pointing back at us.

And when it comes to hormones, I want mine covered by grace and redeemed by wisdom.

So let's talk hormones.

YOUR HORMONAL SYMPHONY

Think of your hormones like a symphony. Each hormone is an instrument with a specific role. When one instrument falls out of tune, the entire performance suffers. For example, insulin regulates blood sugar. When insulin is disrupted, it can lead to insulin resistance and even type 2 diabetes.

Here are some of the key instruments in your body's hormonal orchestra:

- **Insulin**—blood sugar regulation
- **Cortisol**—stress response
- **Estrogen & Progesterone**—female reproductive health
- **Testosterone**—vitality and strength
- **Thyroid hormones**—metabolism and energy
- **Melatonin**—sleep cycles
- **Ghrelin & Leptin**—hunger and fullness

In this chapter, we'll explore the hormones that shape energy, mood, metabolism, and aging in both women and men.

When hormones fall out of balance, life can feel like an orchestra playing without a conductor—loud, chaotic, and exhausting.

But when they are aligned, the body returns to its natural rhythm.

Harmony.
Unity.
Peace.

"I praise you because I am fearfully and wonderfully made."
— Psalm 139:14

Your body was designed with divine precision. The question isn't how God created you. The question is how we steward the temple we've been given.

WHEN YOUR SYMPHONY HITS A SOUR NOTE

Let's be honest.

Hormonal shifts do not send calendar invitations.

They simply arrive.

One day, you are thriving at full tempo. The next day, your inner orchestra sounds like free jazz with no conductor.

Hormones After 40: The Conversation No One Is Having

When people talk about midlife hormone changes, the conversation usually centers around women.

Perimenopause.
Menopause.
Hot flashes.

But men experience hormonal shifts too.
It is called "andropause," or low testosterone.

In other words, this chapter is not just for women.

It is for anyone whose body has ever felt slightly out of rhythm.

Signs the Hormonal Symphony Is Off-Key in Women:

- Irregular periods, hot flashes, or poor sleep
- Low energy, mood swings, anxiety, brain fog, or depression
- Cravings, acne, hair loss, or skin changes
- Breast tenderness or fibrocystic lumps
- Headaches, migraines, or reduced resilience

Signs of Low Testosterone in Men:

- Low libido or erectile dysfunction
- Reduced muscle mass or increased belly fat
- Fatigue or thinning hair
- Irritability, depression, poor focus, or memory changes

Other Signs of Hormonal Imbalance in Men:

- Excess estrogen can cause weight gain, emotional swings, and slower metabolism.
- Excess testosterone can create aggression, acne, sleep disruption, and fluid retention.

And don't forget the supporting players:

- Thyroid hormones influence metabolism, body temperature, and energy.
- Adrenal hormones regulate stress response, stamina, and resilience.

When hormones fall out of tune, everything feels off.

Mind.
Body.
Spirit.

But here is the encouraging truth:

Your hormonal symphony can be tuned again.

Your hormones are not your enemy.
They are your messengers.

With the right habits, you can restore balance, regain energy, and realign your body with the rhythm God designed.

Because you were never meant to live offbeat.

And like any orchestra, the music depends on the instruments.

THE MAIN PLAYERS IN YOUR HORMONAL SYMPHONY

If hormones are the instruments in your body's orchestra, it helps to know who is playing first chair. Like any well-structured ensemble, hormones follow a divine hierarchy. When that order is disrupted, the whole performance suffers.

So let's meet the stars of the show.

Oxytocin—The Conductor of Connection

Oxytocin plays a leading role in the body's connection system. Known as the "love hormone," it's released during hugs, holding hands, childbirth, breastfeeding, prayer, worship, sharing meals, and even petting your dog. It's the glue of emotional bonding, trust, and intimacy.

- Low levels? You might feel disconnected and emotionally flat.
- Too much? Can contribute to mood imbalances.

Cortisol—The Stress Siren

Cortisol is your body's alarm system. It's called the "stress hormone." It revs you up to deal with danger, like facing a tiger or a tax deadline. But when "fight or flight" stays switched on—because of work drama, financial strain, or even the nightly news—your body gets stuck in overdrive.

- Too much cortisol = anxiety, weight gain, low immunity.
- Too little = fatigue and burnout.

Your perspective plays a huge role. Stress isn't always the villain. It's how you view it. Some people panic in traffic. Others turn it into podcast time. Your glass? Half full or half empty? Let's choose full.

Insulin—The Blood Sugar Boss

Produced by the pancreas, insulin helps your cells absorb glucose after meals. It's often called the body's fat-storage hormone because when insulin stays elevated, more fat gets stored.

As Dr. Jason Fung puts it, weight issues are often hormonal, not just about calories in and out.

- Imbalances = insulin resistance, pre-diabetes, diabetes, and energy crashes.
- Balance = better energy, mood, and weight stability.

Estrogen—The Queen of Femininity

Estrogen plays a major role in the glow of health. It helps smooth skin, support hair growth, shape curves, and regulate reproductive health. In both men and women, it helps with bone health and metabolism. Too much or too little in either sex can cause mood swings, fatigue, libido issues, and even cancers.

Progesterone—The Calming Companion

Estrogen's calming counterpart. It calms the mind, balances moods, and supports pregnancy. Dr. Mindy Pelz says it often drops during menopause because of years of stress from our 30s and 40s.

- Low levels = PMS, irregular cycles, anxiety, and fertility issues.
- In men, low progesterone can disrupt testosterone and overall hormonal balance.

Testosterone—The Drive Behind the Dream

Testosterone is often called a "male hormone," but it fuels strength, motivation, and ambition in both men and women.

- Low T in men = fatigue, low libido, muscle loss.
- High T = aggression, acne, sleep issues.

In women, balanced testosterone helps build muscle, boost motivation, and sustain libido. Too much? Think PCOS, facial hair, and irregular cycles.

DHEA—The Master Hormone Builder

DHEA is like the behind-the-scenes stage crew that helps produce progesterone, testosterone, and cortisol. Chronic stress drains it, which throws everything else off.

- Low DHEA = hormonal chaos, especially during menopause.

IS YOUR SYMPHONY IN TUNE?

God designed your hormones to work in harmony. When one player's off, the whole piece sounds messy. But with awareness, stewardship, and a little Kingdom wisdom, you can restore balance, clarity, and peace in your body. Let the healing begin... and the music play on.

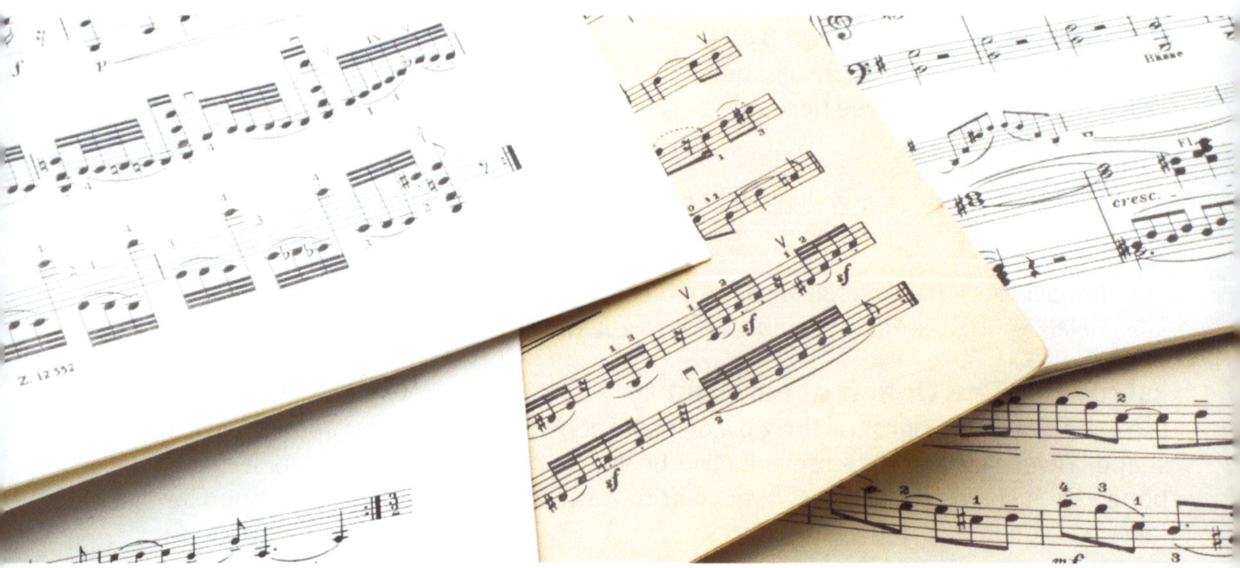

FIVE KEYS TO HAPPY HORMONES

1. ENERGY: Fuel Your Hormones Well

If your energy's crashing by 2 p.m. or you're constantly reaching for caffeine or sugar to power through your day, your hormones are not going to thrive. Insulin plays a leading role in your hormonal symphony.

It's a scientific fact that your sex hormones can't survive a blood sugar rollercoaster. They need stable fuel to function at their best. That's why we use the Fueled for Life Plate Ratio, a simple, sustainable way to keep your blood sugar steady and your energy ueled by fire.

Focus not just on what you put on your plate, but also on the quality, quantity, and frequency of your meals.

If you owned a Ferrari, you wouldn't fill it with cheap fuel. And your body is far more valuable than a car. It's the temple of the Holy Spirit. Let's treat it like royalty.

Quick Nutrition Guide for Hormonal Support:

- **Protein:** Aim for 20g per meal (chicken, fish, eggs, tofu, Greek yogurt, lentils). Your liver needs those amino acids and B vitamins.
- **Cruciferous Veggies:** Broccoli, kale, radishes, cabbage, and spinach support detox pathways. Lightly steam them—your thyroid will thank you.
- **Healthy Fats:** These support bile production and remove toxins. Examples include: nuts, seeds, olive oil, and oily fish (no more than 2x/week to avoid heavy metals), which help with bile flow and hormone clearance.
- **Hydration:** Half your body weight in ounces of water per day. Green tea is a bonus—it supports detox enzymes.
- **Iron & Vitamin C:** When eating iron-rich foods, pair them with vitamin C-rich foods for better absorption. For example, when having a steak, have a salad with it with lemon and herb dressing, followed by a portion of berries.
- **Whole Grains:** B vitamins are needed for detoxification and fiber to support healthy digestion. Examples include: buckwheat, quinoa, and brown rice. Feed your gut and help sweep out waste.

2. GUT HEALTH: Tend the Garden of Your Hormones

Here's a Kingdom secret: your gut isn't just about digestion. It's a command center for your hormones.

Estrogen even has its own support team in your gut called the "estrobolome." These bacteria help regulate estrogen by producing an enzyme called "beta-glucuronidase." When balanced, it properly eliminates used estrogen. But when levels get too high, especially in a sluggish gut, estrogen can be released and returned to circulation.

Think of hormones like a package tied with a bow, ready to leave your body, only to be opened and sent right back inside. That's why we say tend your gut like a garden. A thriving gut creates a thriving hormonal ecosystem.

Signs Your Estrobolome Is Out of Balance (Women):

- Bloating or digestive discomfort
- Acne or skin flare-ups
- Heavy, light, or irregular periods
- Low libido
- Tender or fibrocystic breasts
- Mood swings or irritability
- Hot flashes
- Unexplained weight gain
- PCOS

Steward your gut well, and your hormones, energy, and mood often improve alongside it.

Four P's for Hormone-Supporting Gut Health

- **Probiotics – Beneficial Bacteria** that support digestion and help eliminate excess. Sources include sauerkraut, kimchi, kefir, yogurt, tempeh, miso, fermented vegetables, and cheeses.

- **Prebiotics – Fiber that feeds the healthy bacteria.** These are indigestible fibers that feed healthy bacteria and help them grow. Found in garlic, onions, bananas, and asparagus.

- **Polyphenols – Antioxidant Powerhouses** that reduce inflammation and support gut balance. Found in berries, green tea, dark chocolate, olives, apples, and pomegranates.

- **Phytoestrogens (for women) – Natural plant compounds** that gently support estrogen balance and may reduce symptoms such as hot flashes. Sources include flaxseeds, soy, chickpeas, lentils, sesame seeds, oats, barley, and alfalfa sprouts.

Tip: When increasing fiber or probiotics, start low and go slow. Give your gut time to adjust to avoid unnecessary bloating.

3. CELLULAR SIGNALLING: **Healthy Fats Support Happy Hormones**

Have you ever been on an important phone call when the signal suddenly drops? You can hear the other person trying to speak, but the connection keeps cutting out.

"Hello? Can you hear me now?"

That's exactly what happens in your body when your cells cannot communicate properly. Your hormones are constantly sending messages telling your body what to do. Burn fat. Store energy. Repair tissue. Calm stress. Regulate mood.

Those messages only work if your cells can receive the signal. And that signal travels through your cell membranes, which are made primarily of fat. Think of your cell membrane as the reception tower for your hormones.

When your body has enough healthy fats, those membranes stay flexible and responsive. Signals move clearly from hormone to cell, and your body functions the way it was designed to. But when healthy fats are missing, cell membranes become stiff and sluggish.

Hormone messages start getting lost. Energy drops. Inflammation rises. Metabolism slows. Mood and immunity can suffer.

In other words, the signal gets weak.

Healthy fats help restore that connection. Foods like avocados, nuts, seeds, olive oil, and fatty fish strengthen your cell membranes so hormones can communicate clearly.

Omega-3 fatty acids are especially powerful. They reduce inflammation and help your body properly produce and receive key hormones such as estrogen, testosterone, and insulin. Healthy fats also unlock another important benefit.

They allow your body to absorb the fat-soluble vitamins A, D, E, and K, which support immune health, bone strength, cellular repair, skin clarity, vision, and emotional balance.

When your cells have the right fuel, the signal becomes clear again. And when the signal is clear, your hormones can finally do their job.

Simple Ways to Strengthen Cellular Signaling

- Add avocado or olive oil to meals.
- Eat fatty fish like salmon or sardines twice per week.
- Snack on nuts and seeds instead of processed foods.
- Avoid highly processed vegetable oils that promote inflammation.

Small changes at the table can dramatically improve the way your cells communicate.And when your cells communicate well, your hormones begin to harmonize again.

4. STRESS

Cortisol, your primary stress hormone, plays a major role in your hormonal balance. The problem isn't cortisol itself. It's chronic stress that keeps it elevated and throws the rest of your hormonal symphony out of tune. Unmanaged stress disrupts sleep, affects weight, impacts mood, and can lead to long-term hormone imbalances. This is why your response to stress matters just as much as the stress itself.

Chronic stress is the fastest way to disrupt your hormones.

On the other side of the spectrum is oxytocin, the "love hormone." Oxytocin is a powerful antidote to stress, calming the nervous system and restoring a sense of peace and connection. That's why activities that increase oxytocin, like prayer, worship, physical touch, meaningful conversations, shared meals, and time in God's presence, are not just good for the soul. They're strategic tools for hormonal balance.

Your nervous system needs rhythm, not chaos. And your hormones? They respond to the atmosphere you cultivate. Choose wisely what you allow in—because what you take in emotionally, mentally, and spiritually will show up in your physical output.

When cortisol stays elevated, everything from your mood to your hormones pays the price. Keeping stress in check protects your adrenal glands, and that means better balance for key hormones like estrogen, progesterone, and testosterone.

Strategies to Support a Healthy Stress Response:

- Eat balanced meals that stabilize blood sugar.
- Support gut health.
- Prioritize deep, restorative sleep.
- Spend time outdoors.
- Laugh often and pursue activities that bring joy.
- Cultivate prayer and stillness with God.
- Build strong, supportive relationships.
- Practice daily gratitude.

Science tells us that doing things you love triggers dopamine and endorphins, the natural feel-good chemicals that lower cortisol and help regulate your hormones. But even more than that, Scripture reminds us this is God's design.

Ecclesiastes 3:12-13 says, *"there is nothing better for people than to be happy... eat and drink, and find satisfaction in all their toil—this is the gift of God."*

Joy is not a luxury. It's a Kingdom principle. When you delight in what God has placed in your heart, whether it's music, movement, creativity, or quiet, you realign your body, mind, and spirit with His rhythm for rest and restoration.

5. DETOXIFICATION: Your Liver Is Your Superhero!

Detox isn't about drinking green juice for three days while hoping your headache disappears.

Real detox is much simpler. It's about helping your liver do the job God designed it to do. Every day your body filters toxins, removes what doesn't belong, and restores balance.

Your liver works around the clock to protect your health. But here's the catch. Your results aren't determined only by genetics. They're shaped by how you steward the body you've been given.

Your genetic code is a gift from God, but too many people use genetics as an excuse to keep unhealthy habits.

Genetics may load the gun, but lifestyle pulls the trigger.

Just because diabetes or high blood pressure runs in your family doesn't mean it has to run your future. You didn't inherit the disease. You inherited patterns. And patterns can change.

Detox Is a Traffic Issue

Think of your liver like a highway. Some people are born with a ten-lane highway. Others start with a two-lane country road. That natural capacity is called your "genetic blueprint." But traffic is determined by lifestyle.

When you overload your system with processed food, chemicals, stress, and poor sleep, it's like sending rush hour traffic onto a road that can't handle it. Everything backs up. Instead of blaming your genes, the solution is to manage the traffic by reducing the toxic load your body has to process. When the liver is overloaded, the body begins sending signals.

Signs You Might Need a Detox Tune-Up:

- Hormonal imbalances
- Constipation or acid reflux
- Fatigue, brain fog, or mood swings
- Skin issues such as acne or rosacea
- Sensitivity to smells, alcohol, or caffeine
- Headaches, dizziness, or nausea
- Pain between the shoulder blades or under the ribs

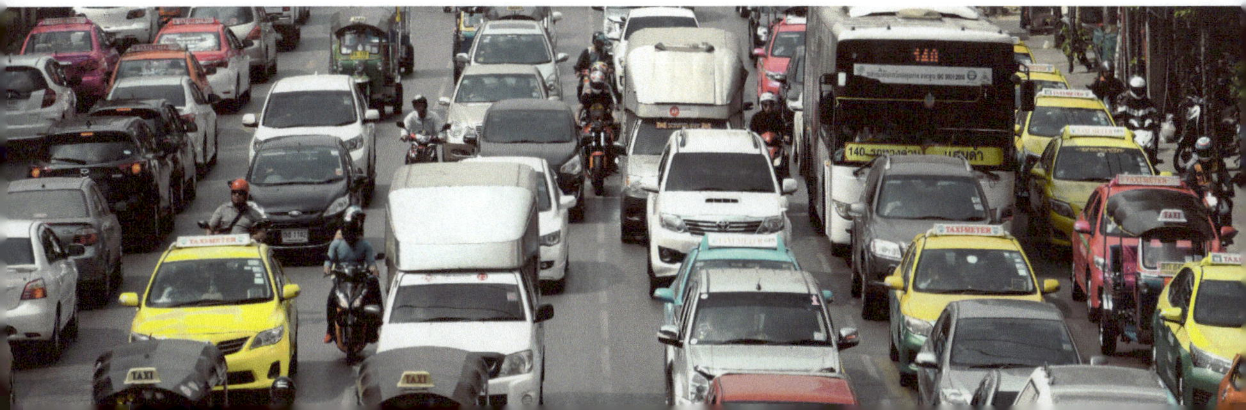

HORMONE HARMONY BLUEPRINT

Five pillars in a quick recap:

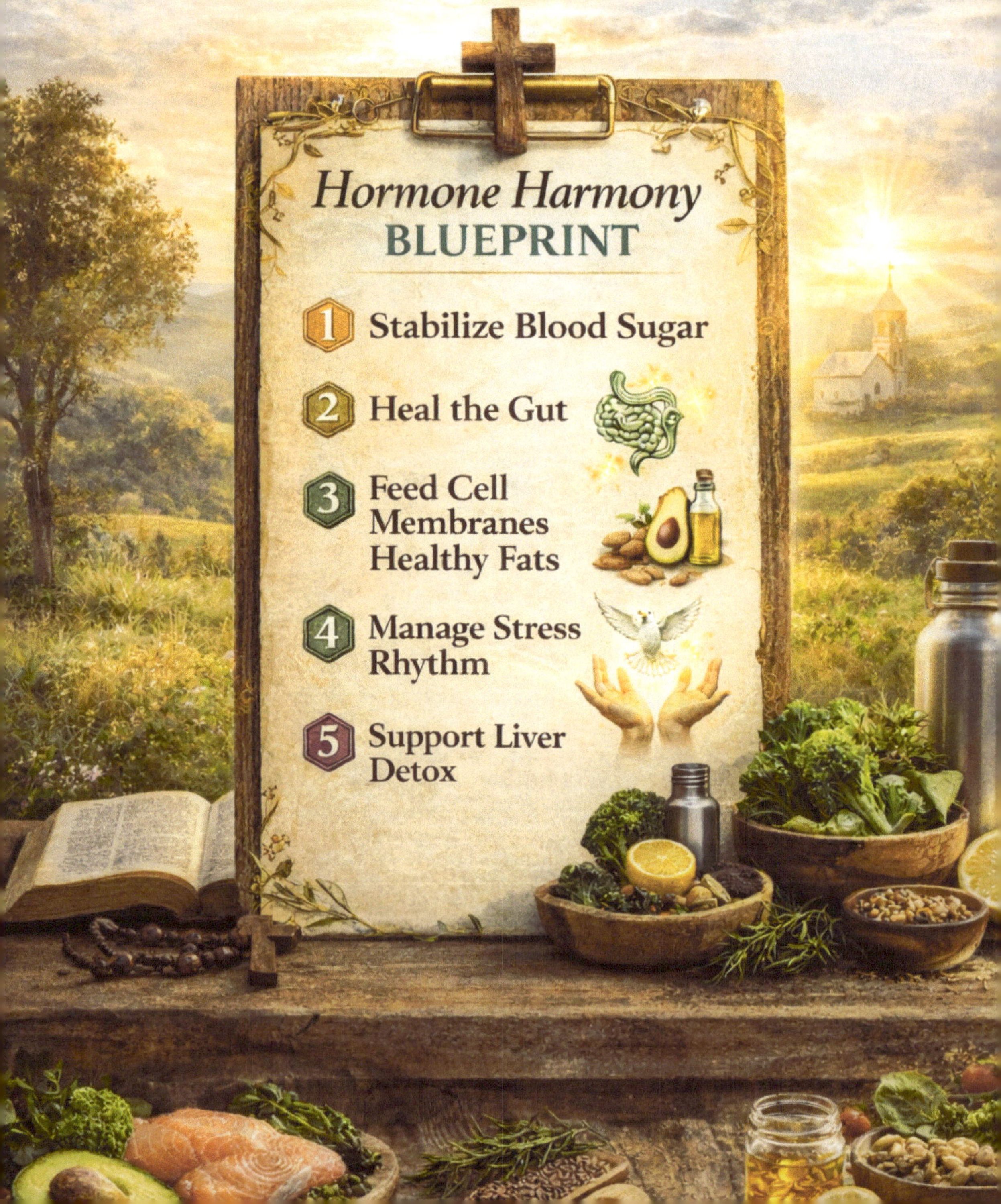

Hormone Harmony
BLUEPRINT
1 Stabilize Blood Sugar
2 Heal the Gut
3 Feed Cell Membranes Healthy Fats
4 Manage Stress Rhythm
5 Support Liver Detox

CHAPTER 12

THE POWER OF FASTING

God's Traffic Controller

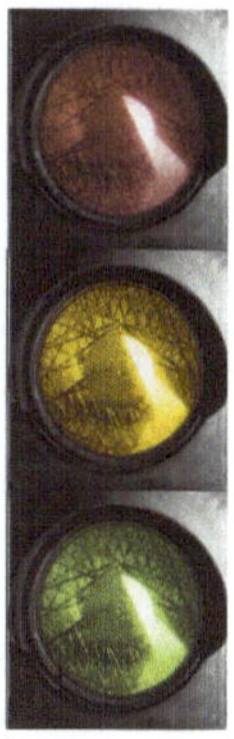

A few years ago, I realized something strange.

Most people are eating all day... and wondering why their bodies never get a chance to heal. They're on a constant roller coaster of trying to heal, but we keep feeding them food that they're trying to detox.

That is why God gave us an incredible piece of wisdom that most people disregard. In fact, think of it like a reset button that most people fail to hit.

What is it? Fasting.

It may be popular in fitness blogs, health podcasts, and biohacking circles, but long before modern science discovered its benefits, God established fasting as Heaven's roadmap for spiritual maturity, physical restoration, detoxification, and Kingdom dominion. It is a major part of His plan to keep your internal traffic clear and moving in harmony with His Spirit.

There's a reason Jesus modeled fasting for His disciples and said:

"When you fast, don't make it obvious, as the hypocrites do, for they try to look miserable and disheveled so people will admire them for their fasting." - Matthew 6:16

Notice—He didn't say "if you fast," but "when you fast."

That one word "WHEN" reveals that fasting was not optional; it was expected.

Fasting is meant to be a habitual rhythm of your spiritual life. It's a private act of devotion that aligns your body, mind, and spirit with God's heart. It's not about earning favor or appearing holy; it's about creating sacred space for intimacy with the Father.

Today, many people fast for physical benefits such as weight loss, gut health, or a metabolic reset. And while those outcomes are real and valuable, they are secondary to God's original design.

Fasting isn't starvation. It's restoration.

Think of your metabolism like a busy intersection. Insulin directs traffic. Hormones send signals. But fasting is the traffic controller that clears the gridlock.

Long before modern science understood metabolic rest and detox pathways, Scripture introduced fasting as a rhythm of renewal for the body and spirit.

Larry's First Fast

I'll never forget Larry's first fast.

This was over thirty years ago, when we were dating.

Larry had just come off the Mr. Oklahoma Bodybuilding Championship. At 6'5" and 275 pounds, he looked exactly like what you'd expect from a former Texas A&M defensive end. Strength was his identity. The gym was his second home.

After college, he moved into sales, but he still trained like a top-tier competitor. Muscle mattered. Performance mattered.

And fasting? That sounded like the worst idea imaginable.

I met Larry at the gym and invited him to a weekly Bible study. That night he gave his life to Christ and stepped into a completely new way of living—one centered on freedom, purity, and purpose. It was also the first time he heard about fasting.

For me, fasting was normal. I had spent years in full-time ministry traveling around the world speaking and serving people. Fasting was part of my rhythm with God. I had done 24-hour fasts, Daniel fasts, and even one 40-day liquid fast. (That kind of fast is not something I recommend unless you know God has specifically called you to it.)

Larry listened to me explain fasting and immediately shook his head.

"I can't do that," he said. "I'll lose muscle. I need every pound I can keep for competition."

That's when we had our first conversation about the difference between starving the body and training the body.

Fasting isn't weakness.
It's discipline.

After a few days of discussion, Larry finally agreed to try a three-day fast.
What happened next surprised everyone.

When he returned to the gym, the other competitors noticed something different. His strength was up. His physique was sharper. His energy was higher.

One of the guys finally asked him, "Larry, what are you doing differently?"

Larry just smiled and winked at me.
He had discovered something powerful.
Fasting wasn't stealing his strength.
It was refining it.

Not long after that season, Larry made an even bigger decision. He stepped away from bodybuilding and chose to pursue God's call on his life. He enrolled in Bible college and began building a career in operations, leadership, and business.

And the gains he experienced from that decision were far greater than muscle.

His spirit grew stronger.
His purpose became clear.
His career flourished.

And along the way, he fell in love with the girl who first introduced him to Jesus... and fasting.

Larry thought fasting would weaken him. Instead, it made him stronger. The same principle applies to your body.

Think of fasting like a holy reset for your body, training it to stop reaching for addictive sugars, drinks, foods, and chemicals that have been wreaking havoc on your organs. When done wisely, fasting helps your body become metabolically flexible. That's just a fancy way of saying it knows how to burn both carbs and fat like a well-oiled, Spirit-led machine.

By lowering insulin resistance, fasting also helps prevent unwanted weight gain and supports better energy, clearer thinking, and yes, more stable moods. It also tackles inflammation, one of the root causes behind hormonal chaos and metabolic mayhem.

Larry thought fasting would weaken him. In reality, fasting activated some of the most powerful healing systems God built into the human body.

Here's How It Works: The Bathtub Detox Model

Your liver detoxes in three phases. Think of it like this: Imagine your body is a bathtub. The water and bubbles in the bathtub are the toxins in your body.

Phase 1: Toxins are temporarily broken down in your bathtub (body) into even nastier forms. Phase 1 is like adding soap to break those toxins down.

Phase 2: Those by-products that are broken down are neutralised and prepped for elimination. Phase 2 is like pulling the plug on the tub.

Phase 3: Elimination - They are excreted in your bile, urine, and stool. Phase 3 is making sure the plumbing isn't clogged. If the drain is blocked, you will get an overflow.

Essentially, fasting allows your body to detoxify the old, dirty, worn-out, non-beneficial toxins, habits, and emotions that have the potential to derail your full potential.

In recent years, some churches have broadened the term fasting to include abstaining from social media, television, or other distractions. While those can be powerful disciplines, true biblical fasting has always centered on withholding food to quiet the flesh, detox the body, and heighten spiritual sensitivity. When you fast from food, you remind your body that your craving stomach is not your master. God is.

In this chapter, we're looking at fasting through the lens of physical health and metabolic restoration. Later in the book, we'll explore fasting the way Jesus practiced it—as a spiritual discipline that realigns the heart with God's voice.

The following fasting rhythms can help reset hormones and restore metabolic balance. When practiced alongside prayer, worship, movement, and healthy nutrition, fasting becomes a powerful tool for both spiritual and physical renewal.

Fasting also improves metabolic flexibility, allowing the body to switch efficiently between fuel sources. This leads to steadier energy, improved fat metabolism, and freedom from constant snacking and energy crashes.

PRACTICAL FASTING RHYTHMS FOR HORMONE RESET

Think of fasting like a rhythm rather than a rule. Different seasons of life may call for different fasting patterns.

SIMPLE FASTING

- **12:12 or 14:10 Intermittent Fasting** - Fast for twelve hours and eat during the following twelve hours each day. Most people already fast every day. It's called sleeping
  - Example: Finish dinner at 7:00 p.m. and eat again at 7:00 a.m.
  - Note: Those with blood sugar issues or taking medications that require food should consult their practitioner.
- **16:8 Intermittent Fasting** - Fast for sixteen hours and eat during an eight-hour window.
  - This deeper rhythm improves insulin sensitivity and shifts the body into fat-burning mode. For men, it may also support testosterone and human growth hormone, which help preserve muscle and energy.
- **20:4 Warrior Fast** - Accelerates fat loss and optimizes insulin sensitivity.

INTERMEDIATE FASTING

- **24-Hour Fasting - (1 to 2x per week)**
  - A powerful spiritual and physical reset. Research has linked periodic twenty-four-hour fasting with improved metabolic flexibility, insulin sensitivity, weight management, and healthy aging.
- **3-Day Water Fast (Monthly or Quarterly)** – A deeper hormonal reset that supports detoxification, cellular repair, and spiritual focus.

THE BIBLICAL "DANIEL" FAST

- **A 21-Day Fast** modeled after the prophet Daniel. This fast focuses on whole foods such as nuts, grains, fruits, vegetables, beans, legumes, and seeds while eliminating animal products, sweeteners, processed foods, and caffeine. Many people experience improvements in skin, inflammation, heart health, and overall body composition during this fast.

Intermittent Fasting for Women During Menstruating Years

A woman's body responds differently to fasting, depending on the day of her cycle. If you are fasting for specific hormonal benefits, consider this:

Menstrual Phase (Days 1–5)

- Estrogen and Progesterone are naturally lower during this phase.
  - Your body is shedding the uterine lining, so energy may be lower.
  - Focus on hydration and iron-rich foods.
  - Practice 12:12 or 14:10 intermittent fasting as listed above.

Follicular (Days 6–14)

- Estrogen is naturally higher in this phase.
  - Best time for a 16:8 or 18:6 intermittent fast.
  - Higher estrogen supports insulin sensitivity and appetite control.
  - Best time for longer fasts, workouts, and lower caloric intake.

Ovulation (Days 14–16)

- Estrogen peaks during this phase.
  - Energy, libido, and metabolic flexibility are higher.
  - Good to include zinc, B vitamins, and ovulation support.
  - Practice the 14:10 or 16:8 intermittent fasting routine.

Luteal (Days 17–24)

- Progesterone is naturally higher during this phase.
  - Reduce to a 12:12 intermittent fast or skip fasting.
  - Progesterone increases your appetite and insulin resistance.

  Focus on blood sugar stability and light meals.

Luteal (Days 25–28)

- Hormone levels naturally decline in this phase.
  - Physical and emotional pre-menstrual symptoms (PMS) could be visible here.
  - Possible mood swings, bloating, cravings, irritability, and fatigue.
  - Body needs more magnesium, carbs, and calories to reduce PMS.
  - Consider stress management and gentle movement.
  - Personalize intermittent fasting according to your body's needs.

Remember: When you learn to fast, you are teaching your body discipline, flexibility, and trust. A body that can fast is a body that is metabolically free.

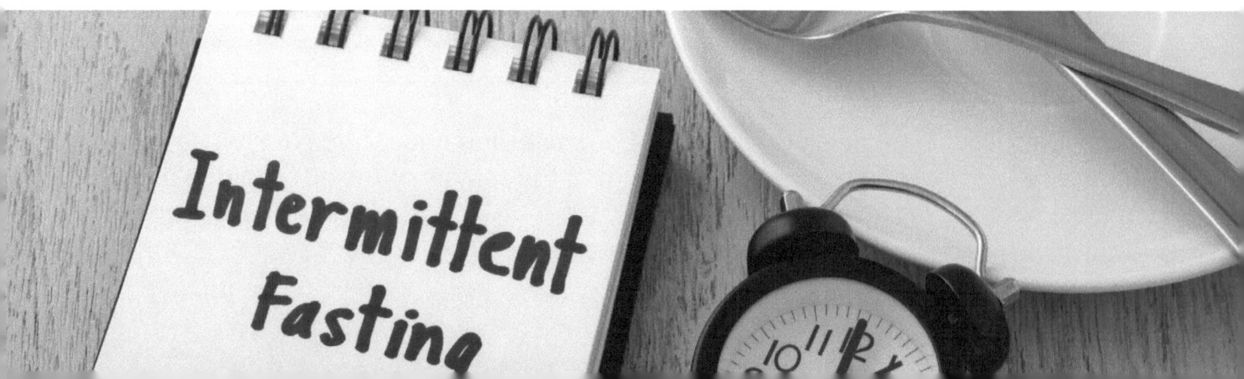

DETOX YOUR HOME

God never designed our bodies to be bombarded with chemicals we can't pronounce. Yet modern living has loaded our homes, clothes, and personal care products with toxins that burden our systems and disrupt our hormones.

- **Textiles & Furniture To Avoid**
  - Flame Retardants – Common in furniture, mattresses, and electronics. Instead, choose organic fabrics and untreated mattresses when possible.
  - PFAS ("forever chemicals") – Found in stain-resistant fabrics and waterproof clothing. Linked to hormone disruption and long-term health concerns. Look for labels that say "PFAS-free" or "flame-retardant-free."
- **Personal Care Products**

Your skin is your largest organ—it absorbs what you apply. Many beauty and hygiene products contain chemicals that act like hormone disruptors, increasing your toxic load without you even knowing.

	What to avoid	**A better solution**
SKINCARE	Parabens, phthalates, synthetic fragrances, formaldehyde	Paraben-free, fragrance-free; natural oils like coconut or shea butter
HAIRCARE	Sulfates (SLS), silicones, artificial dyes	Sulfate- & silicone-free shampoos; apple cider vinegar rinse
MAKEUP	Talc (unless certified asbestos-free), heavy metals, petroleum-based fillers	Clean, mineral-based brands
DEODORANTS	Aluminum, triclosan, synthetic scents	Aluminum-free, naturally scented options
SUNSCREENS	Oxybenzone, octinoxate	Mineral-based with zinc oxide or titanium dioxide
TOOTHPASTE	Triclosan, artificial sweeteners	Natural pastes with baking soda or essential oils
NAIL PRODUCTS	Formaldehyde, toluene, DBP	5-free or 10-free brands; non-acetone removers
PERFUMES & BODY SPRAYS	Synthetic fragrances, phthalates	Essential oil-based or fragrance-free

Clean living isn't about being perfect. It's about being intentional. You are the gatekeeper and steward of your environment. Your body is the temple of the Holy Spirit. When you reduce your toxic load, you free your body to function as God designed it: whole, healthy, and fully alive.

- **Harmful Pesticides and Herbicides**
  - Lawn Care Chemicals: Many contain harmful pesticides. Instead, use natural weed control methods like vinegar or boiling water for a safer lawn care routine.
  - Bug Sprays: DEET-based insect repellents can be harmful with prolonged exposure. For a better solution, choose essential oil-based insect repellents for effective and chemical-free protection.
- **Processed and Packaged Foods**

Forever Chemicals (PFAS): Found in microwave popcorn bags, fast-food wrappers, and takeout containers, these chemicals can leach into food. Instead, make popcorn at home using organic kernels and stovetop methods for a healthier snack.

Minimize consumption of fast food and packaged snacks to reduce exposure to harmful packaging materials. By making informed choices about the products we use and consume, we can significantly reduce our exposure to harmful chemicals and create a healthier environment for ourselves and future generations.

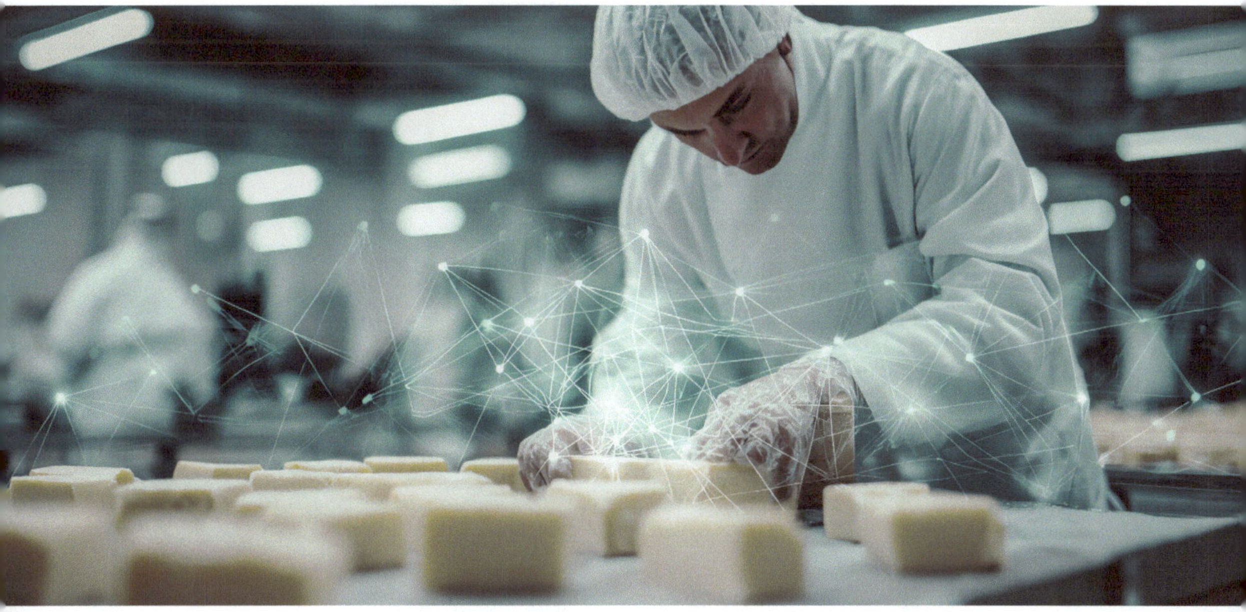

HELPFUL APPS TO IDENTIFY CLEAN PRODUCTS:

1. **Yuka:** Provides detailed analyses of personal care and food products, rating them on safety and suggesting better options.
2. **Think Dirty:** Scan product barcodes to see a toxicity rating and find safer alternatives.

PILLAR 5: MOVEMENT

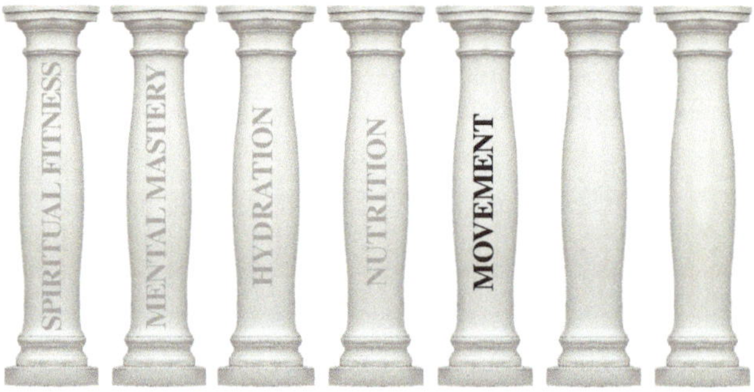

"Therefore I do not run like someone running aimlessly. I do not fight like a boxer beating the air. I discipline my body and bring it under control so that after preaching to others, I myself will not be disqualified for the prize."

— 1 Corinthians 9:26-27

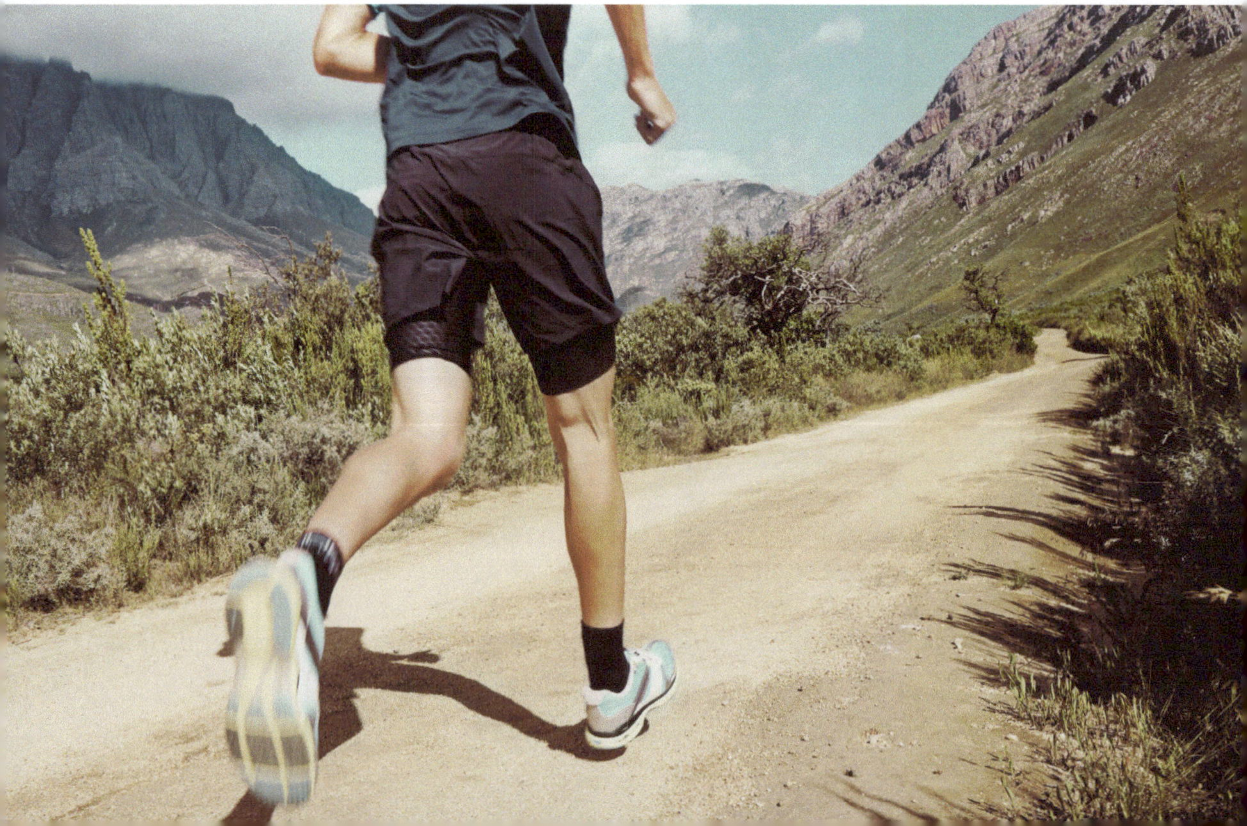

CHAPTER 13
INTENTIONAL EXERCISE

Movement With a Purpose

You don't have to be a professional athlete to pursue peak performance. Scripture makes it clear that caring for your body, the temple God entrusted to you, is an act of worship.

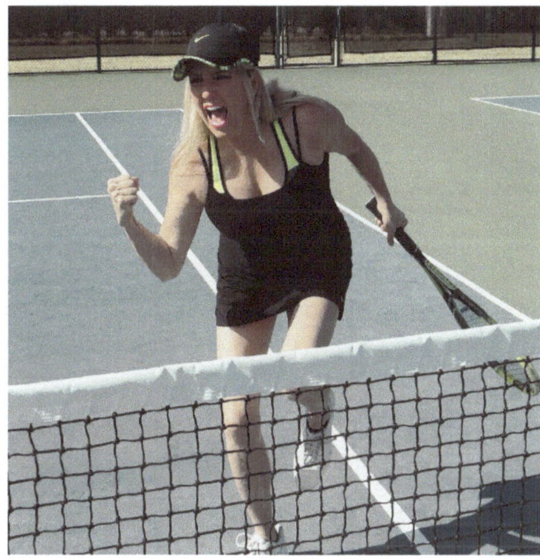

"Therefore, I urge you, brothers and sisters, in view of God's mercy, to offer your bodies as a living sacrifice, holy and pleasing to God. This is your true and proper worship."
— Romans 12:1

In this pillar, we'll focus on a simple question: How do you begin moving your body with intention?

THE 1% METHOD OF MICRO-PROGRESS

From this day forward, the goal is simple: one percent better movement each day.

Instead of chasing a massive fitness overhaul, start with small, consistent shifts. Park at the back of the parking lot instead of near the door. Take a walk during lunch instead of sitting at your desk. Go for a brisk walk after dinner. Even doing household chores with intention can increase your daily movement.

Small actions compound. Within days, you'll notice clearer thinking, better energy, and a growing sense of momentum.

Walking is one of the simplest and most powerful ways to improve your health. Unlike fat, muscle is metabolically active, meaning it burns calories even at rest.

Regular walking helps preserve lean muscle while supporting healthy weight loss and metabolic stability.

LET'S MOVE

Your body was never designed to sit idle. It was created to move—with strength, purpose, and rhythm. Exercise isn't just about burning calories or chasing a number on a scale. It's about stewarding the body God entrusted to you and aligning your life with the energy you were created to live with.

Movement is one of the most powerful activators of hormonal balance. When done wisely and consistently, it boosts testosterone in men, helping build strength, stamina, and confidence. For women, it supports the beautiful interplay between estrogen and progesterone, essential for fertility, regular cycles, and emotional resilience.

Exercise also reduces cortisol, improves insulin sensitivity, and enhances circulation. These shifts help bring your body back into balance. The result? Better energy, deeper sleep, improved mood, stronger relationships, and greater vitality.

This pillar isn't about perfection. It's about intention. Whether you lift weights, walk outside, dance in your living room, or stretch in quiet prayer—every movement matters.

It's Time to Get Active

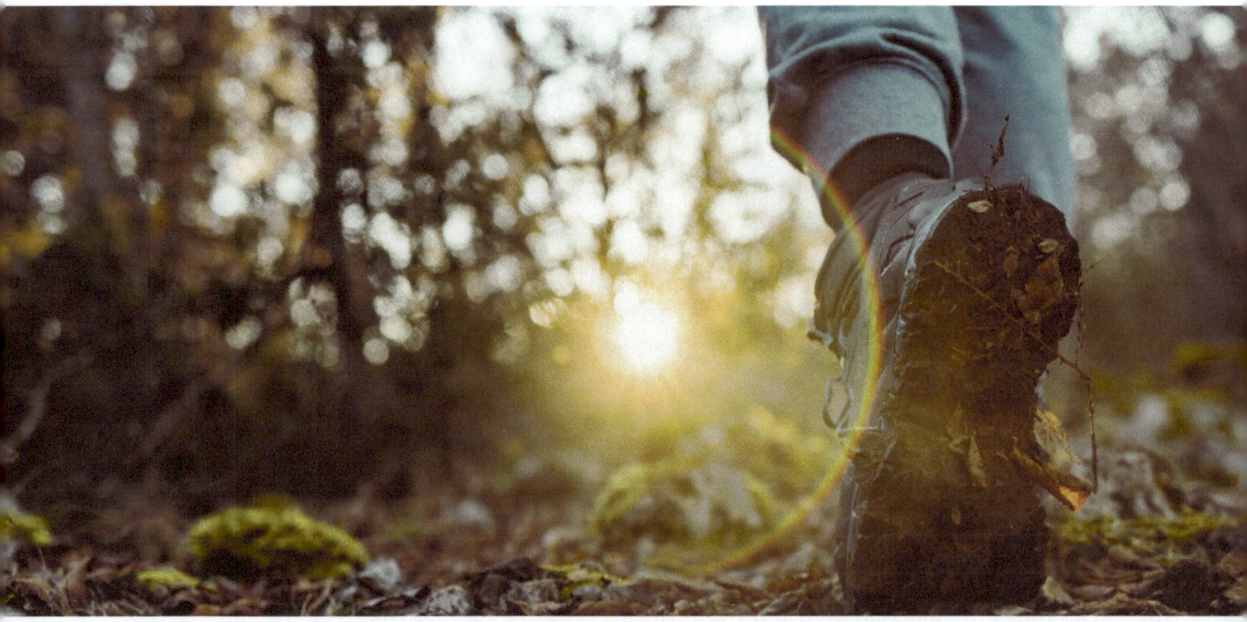

Maintaining muscle mass is key to sustaining long-term results. Walking not only aids fat burning but also helps combat age-related muscle decline, helping you retain strength and muscle function as you age. In essence, regular walking can enhance your metabolic rate, making it easier to maintain a healthy weight while promoting overall wellness.

An example from nature could be the process of photosynthesis in trees. Just as trees rely on consistent sunlight to fuel their growth and maintain a healthy system, walking provides your body with the steady, daily movement it needs to fuel fat-burning and maintain muscle.

Like leaves capturing light to create energy, each step you take ignites your muscles, which in turn helps burn calories more efficiently. And just as trees grow stronger with time and consistent nourishment, your muscles and metabolism thrive when regularly "fed" by movement, making it easier to sustain your weight loss and overall health for years to come.

FOUR REASONS TO WALK AFTER MEALS

Improved Digestion
Walking stimulates digestion and helps move food through the stomach and intestines, reducing bloating and discomfort.

Blood Sugar Regulation
A short walk after meals helps your muscles use glucose for energy, lowering post-meal blood sugar spikes and supporting metabolic health.

Enhanced Metabolism
Movement after eating increases metabolic activity, helping your body burn calories more efficiently.

Reduced Stress
Light physical activity lowers cortisol and promotes relaxation, helping prevent the sluggish feeling that often follows a large meal.

Let's start with the basics.

Write down three ways you will intentionally move your body today.

1. ______________________________

2. ______________________________

3. ______________________________

This week, make it a point to do one or all of the activities you listed here. This will add 20-30 minutes of additional physical exercise to your time-blocking. No matter what level of fitness you are at, increase it by 20-30 minutes of new physical exertion or intensity.

ELEVATE YOUR INTENSITY

When life gets busy, exercise is usually the first thing we abandon.

What we don't realize is that our physical activity stimulates endorphins and oxygen flow which could be a significant key to our decision-making abilities, our attitude, our emotional discipline, and more. When we forgo fitness, we forgo living our best life.

This week, aim for 1% progress.

If you're new to exercise, start with 20–30 minutes of activity at a moderate effort level of 3–5 on a scale of 0–10. Level 0 feels like sitting on the couch. Level 4 might feel like a brisk walk where you can still talk, but you're slightly winded.

Even if you're not a beginner, moderate exertion is important because this is where your body becomes most efficient at burning fat for fuel. At an exertion level of about 4–6, your metabolism relies more heavily on fat as its primary energy source.

When intensity climbs too high, your body shifts toward burning stored carbohydrates, essentially the energy from your most recent meals.

The goal is to train your body to become efficient at burning fat consistently, not just the calories you recently consumed.

Everyone, regardless of shape, size, or genetic makeup, has 119 hours of stored fat to use as an energy source.

Heart rate training (interval training, monitoring your heart rate) will help you burn more fat and make exercise more enjoyable. Rather than trying to exercise hard, exercise smart. When you exercise hard, you are probably just using up depleted carbs (sugar). By exercising smartly, you are burning fat, which will ultimately help you reach your goal a lot faster!

Many fitness plans push long hours in the gym. But the most sustainable approach is consistent, moderate movement that strengthens your heart and can be maintained for life.

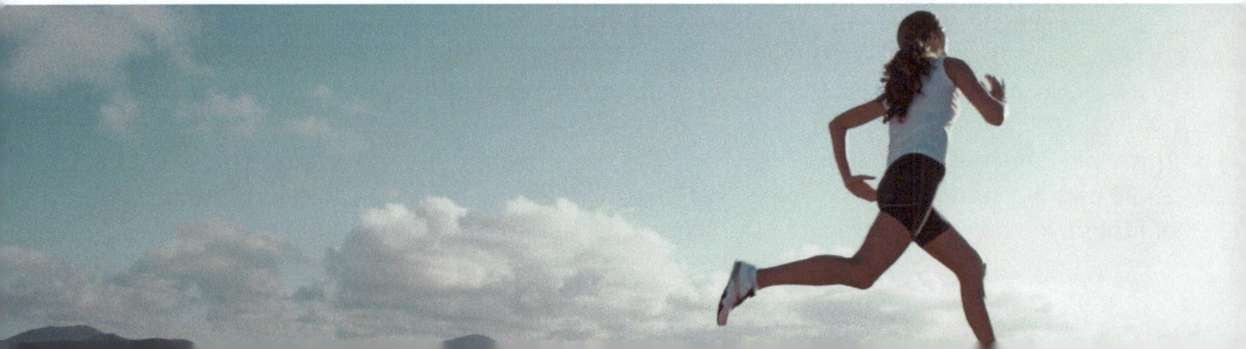

BURN FAT NOT SUGAR!

Many people believe the key to losing weight is working out longer and harder. If they aren't sweaty, exhausted, or sore afterward, they assume the workout didn't count.

But that belief is one of the biggest misconceptions in fitness.

The truth is that your body has a specific metabolic zone where it becomes most efficient at burning fat for fuel. When you understand how to train in that zone, you can work smarter instead of harder and achieve far better long-term results.

Have you ever exercised consistently but still struggled to lose weight?

If so, you may be missing an important principle built into the way God designed your body. Our bodies were never meant to run endlessly at extreme intensity. Nor were they designed to depend on stimulants or artificial performance boosters.

Instead, your body functions like a remarkably intelligent machine operating most efficiently under specific conditions.

Modern exercise science has shown that this optimal efficiency can be identified through heart-rate training. By exercising within a specific heart-rate range, your body learns to rely more heavily on fat for fuel rather than burning the carbohydrates from your most recent meal.

This is called the "fat-burning zone."

What Is A Fat Burning Zone?

Your fat-burning zone is the level of exertion where your body primarily uses stored fat as fuel rather than carbohydrates.

If your goal is to reduce body fat and improve metabolic health, the majority of your workouts should occur in this zone. In fact, research suggests that about eighty percent of your exercise should stay within your fat-burning range.

To identify your fat-burning zone, we need to estimate something called your "anabolic threshold" (AT).

Your anabolic threshold is the point at which your body begins shifting from burning fat to burning carbohydrates for fuel. When your heart rate rises above this level, your body increasingly relies on sugar rather than fat.

Since our goal is to burn fat efficiently, most of our workouts should remain below this threshold.

Every person's fat-burning zone is slightly different. That's why one-size-fits-all workout plans rarely work long term.

Instead, we want to identify the heart-rate range where your body performs most efficiently. A simple 30-minute test can help estimate this range.

During this test, you will exercise for 30 minutes at the highest effort you can comfortably sustain. Your average heart rate during the final 20 minutes will help estimate your anabolic threshold and guide your ideal training zones.

Note: We recommend that you do NOT perform this test alone, but have a partner with you to keep track of your numbers. As with all exercise programs, we strongly suggest getting a doctor's clearance and approval before beginning any type of exercise.

THE ZONE HEART RATE TEST

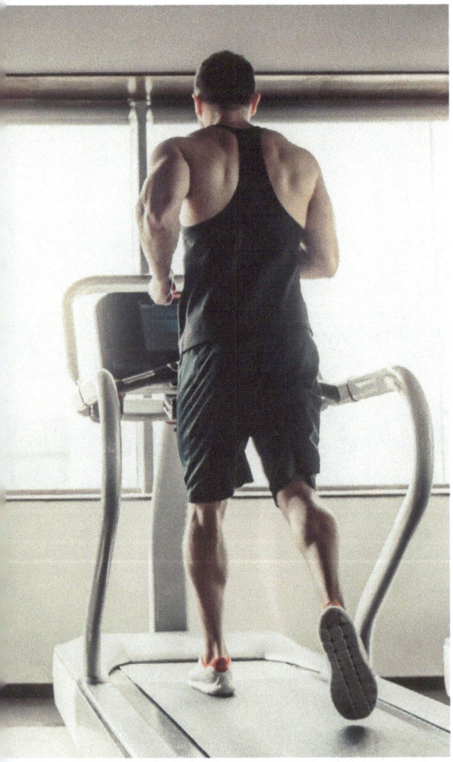

You can perform this 30-minute test using walking, running, cycling, or another endurance activity. A treadmill or stationary bike works especially well because it allows you to monitor your heart rate easily.

Use a heart-rate monitor if possible, or the sensors commonly available on gym equipment.

Step One: Warm up and stretch for 10 minutes at a comfortable pace.

Step Two: Gradually increase your effort until you reach the highest pace you can sustain for 20 minutes.

Step Three: Record your heart rate every minute during those 20 minutes.

Step Four: Add those numbers together and divide by 20. This gives you your average heart rate, which estimates your anabolic threshold.

This average number represents your estimated anabolic threshold. Above this level, your body begins relying more heavily on carbohydrates instead of fat.

Ideally, your fat-burning workouts should stay 10–20 beats below this threshold.

For example, if your threshold is 160 beats per minute, your fat-burning zone would likely fall around 140–150 bpm.

If you don't have access to heart-rate equipment, there is another simple way to measure exercise intensity.

It's called the Borg Rating of Perceived Exertion (RPE) scale.

Instead of measuring heart rate, this method measures how the exercise feels on a scale from 0 to 10. A 0 represents no exertion—like sitting in a chair. A 10 represents maximum effort, where you cannot sustain the pace for long.

For 3 days a week, keep your intensity in your fat-burning zone for 80% of your training time with an exertion level of 3-6 (Zone 1-2).

BORG RPE SCALE
RATED PERCEIVED EXERTION

ZONE 1: Recovery
0 - No exertion at all
1 - Very light
2 - Light

ZONE 2: Fat Burning
3 – Moderate effort (easy activity)
4 – Slightly winded but comfortable
5 – Breathing heavier but still able to talk
6 – Near the edge of the conversation zone

ZONE 3: High Intensity
7 – Hard effort
8 – Very hard cardio
9 – Near maximum effort
10 – Total fatigue

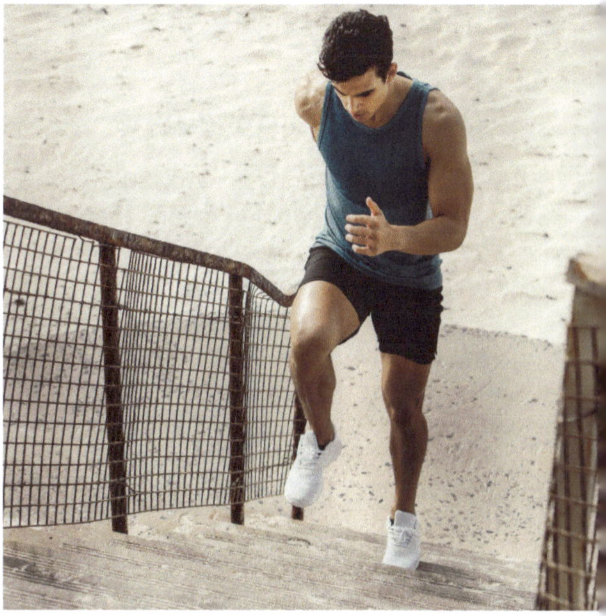

THE TALK TEST

ZONE 1-2: This is like walking with a friend but still able to carry on a conversation. In zones 1 and 2, you might be slightly winded, but not exhausted.

ZONE 3: 2 times per week, go ahead and push yourself to Zone 3 (an exertion level of 7-8). Those will be your cardio health days. At a level 7-8, you should not be able to talk freely due to the level of exertion.

To maintain a balanced fitness routine, alternate workouts across Zones 1, 2, and 3. The specific exercise you choose is less important than the intensity level. Walking, running, cycling, swimming, aerobics, and strength circuits can all work effectively.

THE
FAT-BURNING RULE

Most people exercise too hard to burn fat.

Low Intensity → FAT
Moderate Intensity → FAT + SUGAR
High Intensity → SUGAR

"80% of your workouts should stay in the fat-burning zone."

ZONE TRAINING

ZONE 1: Fat Burning Zone

Workout in Zone 1 for 30-60 minutes. This would mean that you could carry on a meaningful conversation the entire time, despite being slightly winded. It should be a long, steady exercise that is not too strenuous. Your body will be burning fat efficiently and working comfortably. So, for example, if your AP (anabolic threshold) is 160 bpm, then, on these days, you need to keep your heart around 130-140 bpm.

3 Days Per Week

Minutes	Rate of Intensity (ZONE 1)
1-5	3
6-10	4
11-15	5
16-18	3
19-22	4
23-25	5
26-30	3

ZONE 2: Fat Burning Zone

Train in Zone 2 for 30–60 minutes at a moderate intensity. This level builds endurance while teaching your body to burn fat more efficiently.

You should feel slightly challenged but still able to maintain the workout without excessive strain.

For example, if your anabolic threshold is 160 bpm, your Zone 2 training would typically fall between 140–150 bpm.

One Day Per Week

Minutes	Rate of Intensity (ZONE 2)
1-5	3
6-10	4
11-14	5
15-17	6
18-22	5
23-27	4
28-30	3

The secret to sustainable fat loss isn't exercising harder. It's learning how to burn fat instead of sugar.

ZONE 3: (Sugar Burning Zone)

Zone 3 workouts elevate your heart rate and strengthen cardiovascular performance. These sessions are more demanding and should be performed less frequently.

During the higher-intensity intervals, conversations become difficult.

If your anabolic threshold is 160 bpm, these workouts may push your heart rate into the 160–170 bpm range.

One Day Per Week:

Minutes	Rate of Intensity (ZONE 3)
1-5	3-5
6-10	7-8
11-13	3-5
14-18	7-8
19-21	3-5
22-26	7-8
27-30	3-5

PILLAR 6:
REST

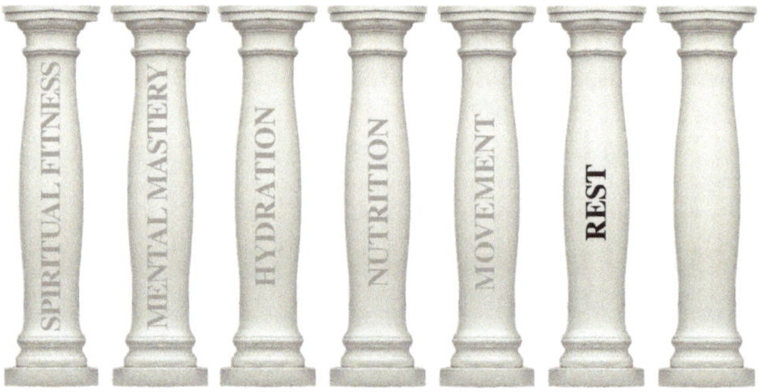

"In vain you rise early and stay up late, toiling for food to eat, for he grants sleep to those he loves."
— Psalm 127:2

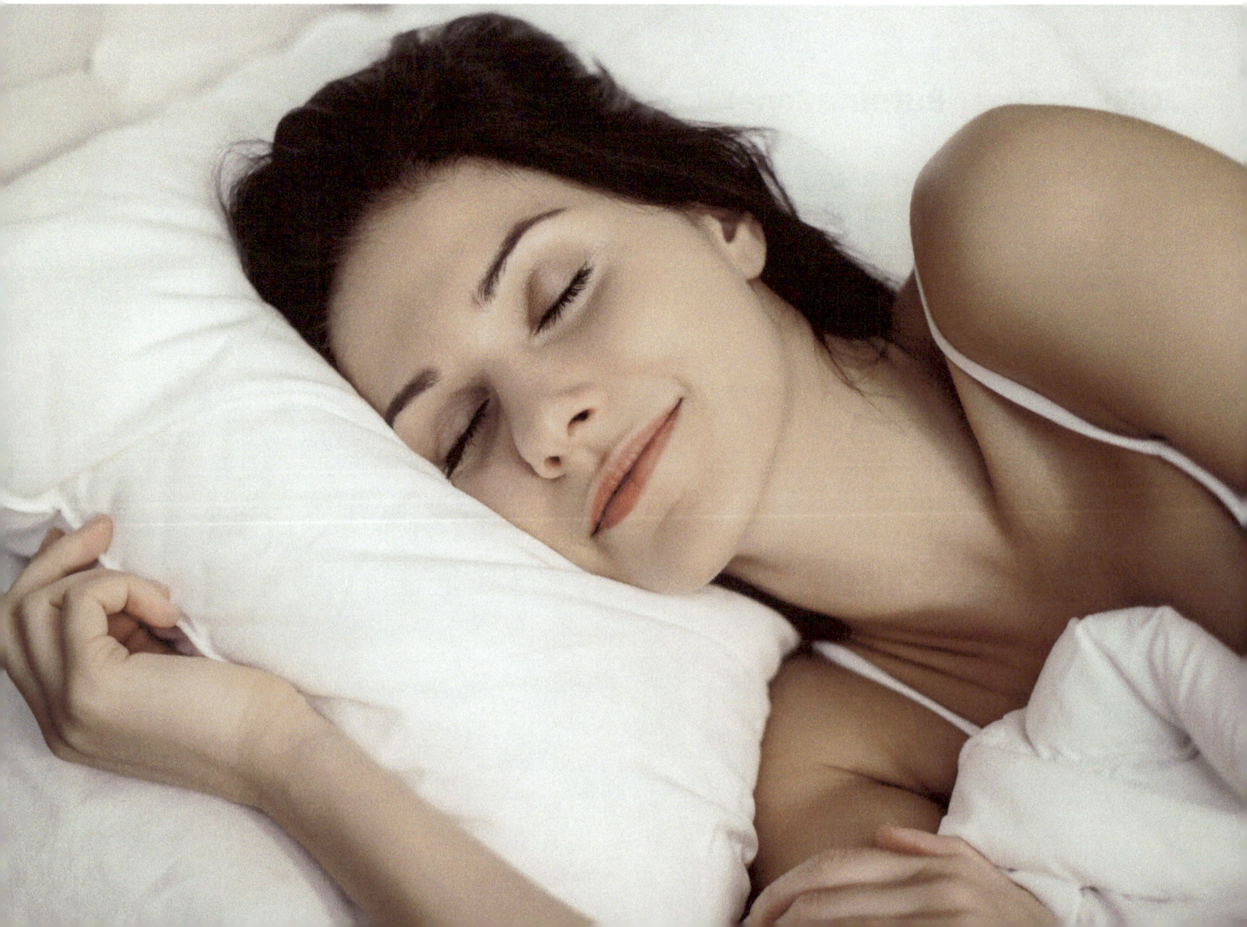

CHAPTER 14

REST IS NOT A LUXURY

IT'S A KINGDOM STRATEGY

God Created You to Function Best with Rest

We live in a world obsessed with more.

More noise.
More hustle.
More consumption.
More pressure to keep pushing forward.

Billions of dollars are spent convincing us that rest is weakness and that productivity requires constant motion. Yet, no matter how much we feed the flesh, our souls remain weary.

Why?

Because what we truly need is rest, stillness, and intentional pause. We need moments that recalibrate our lives and realign us with God's rhythm.

OVERFED YET UNDERNOURISHED

Not long ago, I was standing in a bookstore when the closing announcement echoed through the aisles. As I checked out, the clerk smiled and said, "Now the real work begins."

She explained that once the last customer leaves, the staff restocks the shelves and prepares the store for the next day.

That image stayed with me because your body works the same way.

At the end of each day, your body needs to "close the doors."

During sleep, your body restocks energy, repairs cells, restores organs, calms the nervous system, and resets the mind.

Sleep is not simply rest.
It is restoration.

If you keep pushing without allowing your body time to recover, your system will eventually force you to stop, often through burnout, illness, or emotional breakdown.

True wellness requires Sabbath for the soul and sleep for the body.

Don't wait for a breakdown to make rest a priority. Let God lead you into His rhythm, where restoration becomes your strength.

Fatigue has quietly become a national epidemic.

To keep up with the pace of modern life, people rely on energy drinks, stimulants, sugary foods, sleeping pills, and antidepressants. Every day we pour chemicals into our bodies just to maintain a level of functioning that once came naturally.

Over time, this becomes a cycle.

Stimulants push us forward during the day.
Sedatives pull us down at night.

The result is a biochemical roller coaster that leaves many people feeling exhausted, anxious, and mentally depleted.

The good news is that you can take authority over your health by giving your body the intentional pauses it was designed to receive. Quality sleep and intentional rest restore the body, renew mental clarity, and strengthen your ability to make wise decisions throughout the day.

THE FOUR STAGES OF SLEEP

There was a time when I used to brag about needing only four hours of sleep each night. That was before I understood the critical role sleep plays in metabolism, hormone balance, brain health, and long-term wellness.

Neuroscientist Matthew Walker, author of *Why We Sleep*, explains it simply: *"The shorter your sleep, the shorter your life."*

Sleep allows the brain and body to shift into repair mode. When we consistently miss out on deep sleep, those recovery processes are interrupted, affecting mood, energy, metabolism, memory, and long-term health.

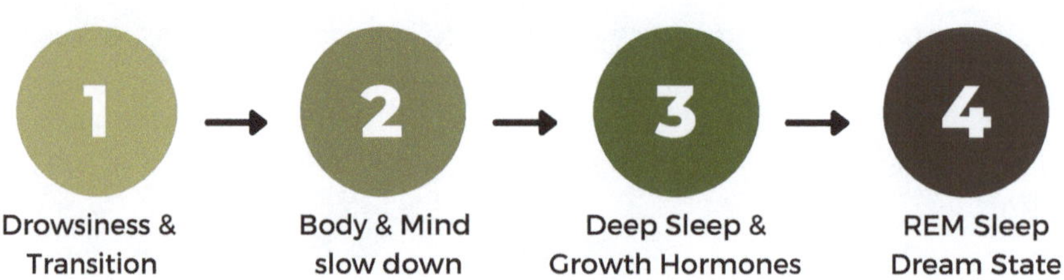

Like water, food, oxygen, and fasting, sleep is not an optional activity in life. It is a MANDATORY function of long life, hormonal balance, internal peace, and optimal wellness.

Did you know that if you get less than seven hours of sleep each night or greater than nine hours, you increase your risk of cancer, heart disease, diabetes, obesity, and other degenerative diseases? According to research, being able to go into a deep, dreamless sleep zone can even help to regulate your metabolism. That is GREAT news for anyone wanting to lose weight or restore their health.

The first three stages of sleep are called non-REM sleep.

Stage One - Drowsiness
This is the brief transition between wakefulness and sleep. Your body begins slowing down and drifting into rest.

Stage Two - Light Sleep
Your body temperature drops, your heart rate slows, and the brain prepares for deeper sleep.

Stage Three - Deep Sleep
This is the most restorative stage of sleep. The body repairs tissues, strengthens the immune system, and restores physical energy.

Stage Four - REM Sleep
REM sleep is the dreaming stage. Brain activity increases while the body remains still, helping process memories, emotions, and learning.

Deep sleep regulates critical hormones.

Just two nights of poor sleep can lower leptin (the hormone that signals fullness) by twenty percent while increasing ghrelin (the hunger hormone) by thirty percent. In other words, lack of sleep literally makes you hungrier and less satisfied—a powerful disadvantage for anyone trying to maintain a healthy weight.

Stages three and four are the most restorative phases of sleep, helping you think clearly, feel energized, and wake refreshed.

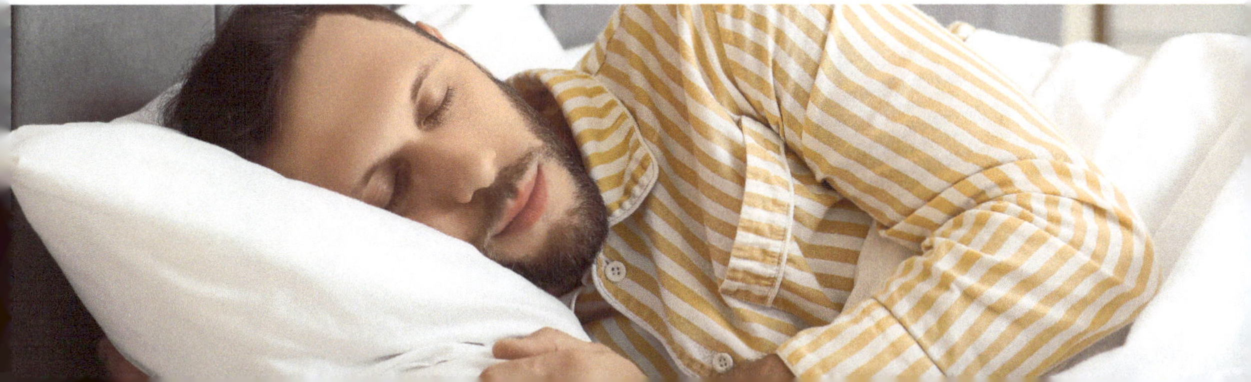

7 DANGERS OF SLEEP DEPRIVATION

1. **SICKNESS**
   Lack of sleep weakens the immune system. Research shows that people who sleep fewer than seven hours per night are significantly more vulnerable to infections, including the common cold.

2. **DISEASE**
   Chronic sleep deprivation increases the risk of high blood pressure, diabetes, obesity, heart disease, and stroke.

3. **LETHARGY**
   Sleep loss slows reaction time, reduces focus, and impairs coordination, leaving you feeling mentally foggy and physically drained.

4. **INCONSISTENCY**
   Sleep deprivation harms workplace performance and productivity. In the United States alone, poor sleep costs the economy billions of dollars each year.

5. **IRRESPONSIBILITY**
   Drowsy driving is responsible for over 100,000 crashes each year and thousands of fatalities.

6. **IMPOTENCE**
   Lack of sleep disrupts hormone production and can significantly lower testosterone levels and sexual health.

7. **CRITICAL THINKING**
   Poor sleep reduces attention span, decision-making ability, emotional regulation, and mental clarity.

Even losing one hour of sleep can impair cognitive performance.

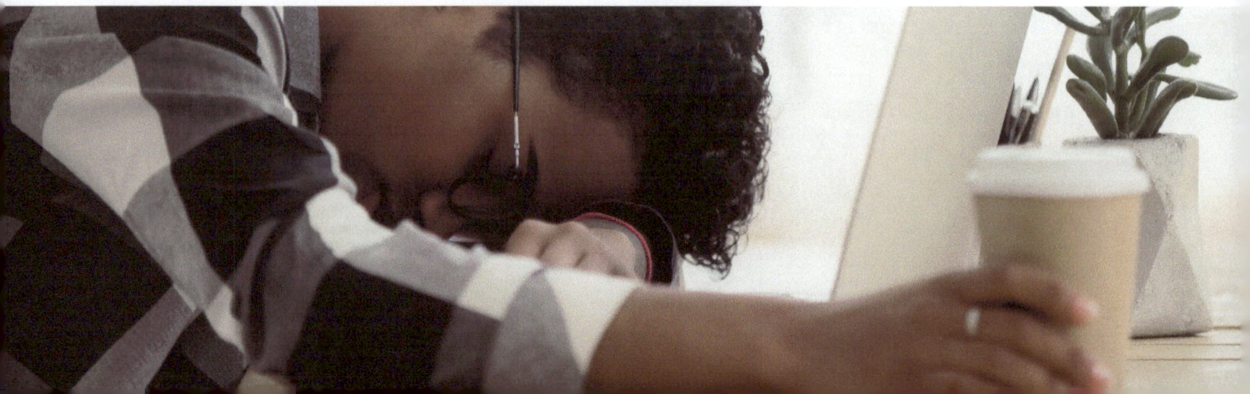

10 WAYS TO CREATE THE BEST SLEEP ENVIRONMENT

1. **DIM THE LIGHTS**
   Light regulates your body's internal clock, known as the "circadian rhythm." Expose yourself to natural light in the morning and reduce artificial and blue light in the evening. Watching the sunrise and sunset helps reset your biological clock. A quality sleep mask can also improve sleep quality.

2. **COMFORTABLE MATTRESS AND PILLOW**
   Your mattress and pillow should support proper spinal alignment. Choose bedding that supports your body and keeps your neck and head comfortably aligned.

3. **MAINTAIN A COOL TEMPERATURE**
   The ideal bedroom temperature for sleep is typically 65–68°F (18–20°C). Experiment to find the temperature at which your body sleeps best.

4. **BLOCK OUT NOISE**
   Noise disrupts deep sleep. Use white noise, earplugs, or noise-canceling devices to minimize external sounds.

5. **BANISH ELECTRONICS FROM THE BEDROOM**
   Phones, tablets, and computers emit blue light that suppresses melatonin, the hormone responsible for sleep. Replace evening screen time with reading, journaling, or quiet reflection.

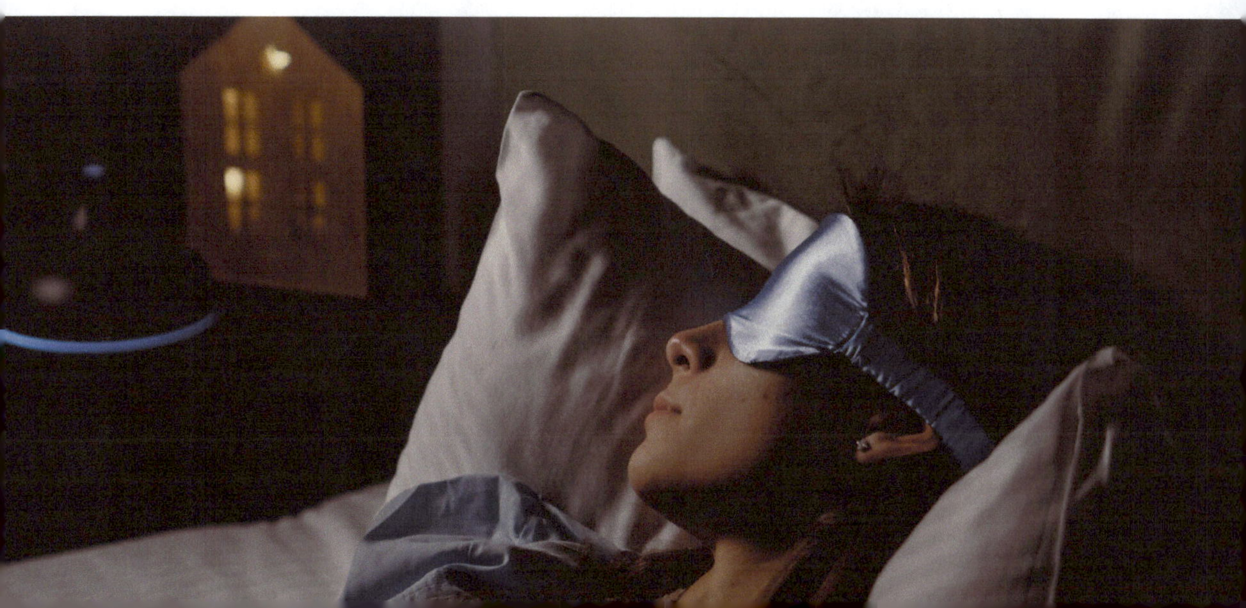

6. **CHOOSE CALMING COLORS**
   Your bedroom environment affects how quickly your body relaxes. Soft blues, gentle greens, and muted earth tones promote calm. Avoid bright or overly stimulating colors.

7. **CREATE A CLUTTER-FREE SPACE**
   A cluttered room often leads to a cluttered mind. Keep your sleep environment clean, organized, and peaceful.

8. **DEVELOP A RELAXING BEDTIME ROUTINE**
   Create a consistent evening rhythm—reading, stretching, prayer, or a warm bath. When repeated nightly, these cues train your body to prepare for sleep.

9. **INCORPORATE NATURAL ELEMENTS**
   Nature calms the nervous system. Consider plants, natural textures, or calming artwork to create a peaceful environment.

10. **USE A HEPA AIR FILTER**
    Clean air supports deeper sleep. HEPA filters remove dust, pollen, allergens, and airborne irritants that can interfere with rest.

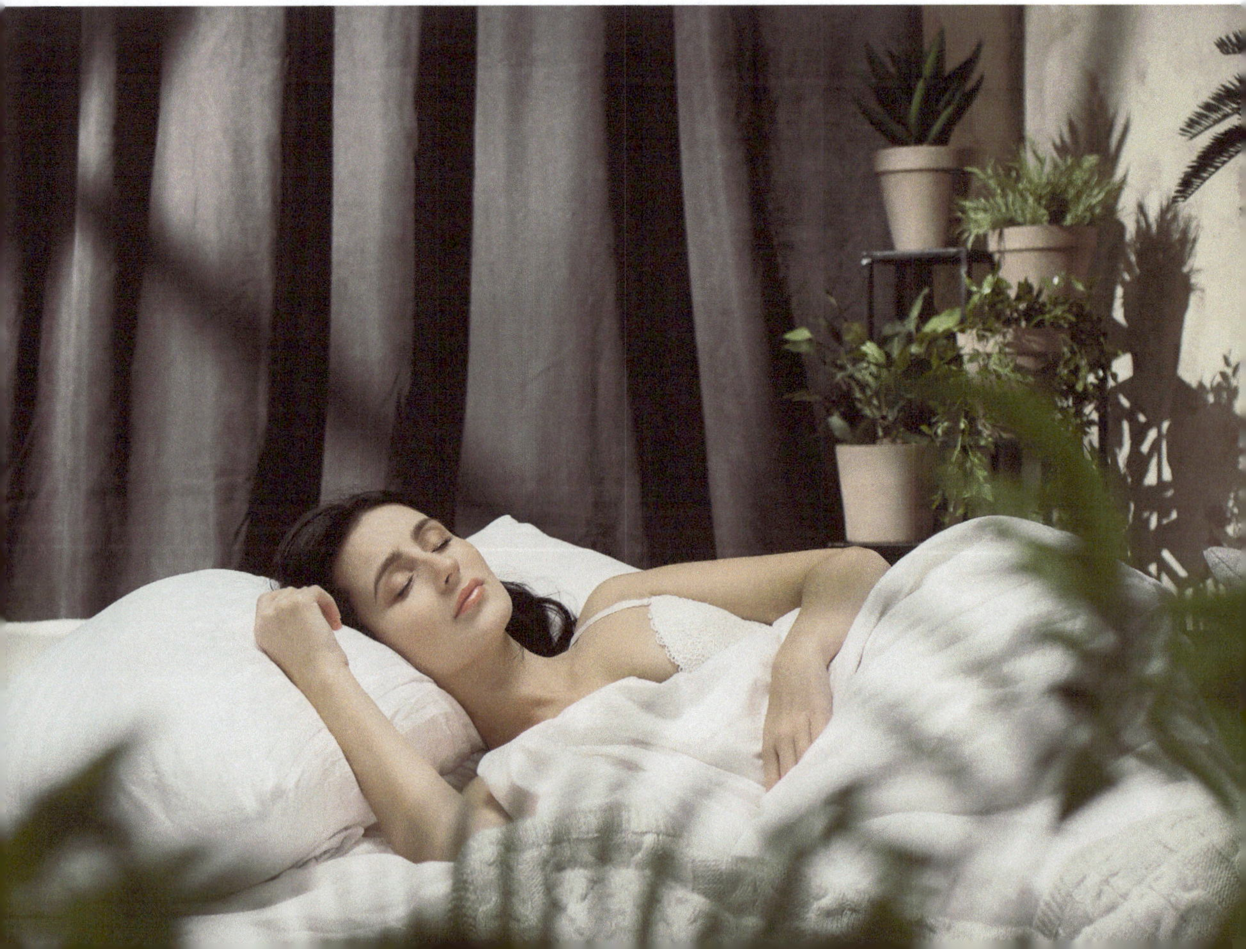

15 NATURAL SUPPLEMENTS THAT SUPPORT DEEP, RESTORATIVE SLEEP

1. **VALERIAN ROOT**
   Traditionally used to promote relaxation and help with falling asleep.

2. **CHAMOMILE**
   Often consumed as tea. Contains compounds that promote calm and relaxation.

3. **LAVENDER**
   Known for its soothing aroma. Often used in aromatherapy or pillow sprays.

4. **PASSIONFLOWER**
   Supports relaxation by increasing GABA activity in the brain.

5. **LEMON BALM**
   A gentle herb traditionally used to reduce anxiety and promote restful sleep.

6. **ASHWAGANDHA**
   An adaptogenic herb that helps the body manage stress, indirectly improving sleep quality.

7. **MAGNOLIA BARK**
   May reduce anxiety and support deeper sleep.

8. **MELATONIN**
   The hormone that regulates your sleep-wake cycle. Supplements may help regulate sleep patterns, especially during travel or schedule disruptions.

9. **MAGNESIUM GLYCINATE**
   Supports nervous system relaxation and muscle recovery.

10. **L-THEANINE**
    An amino acid found in green tea that promotes calm without sedation.

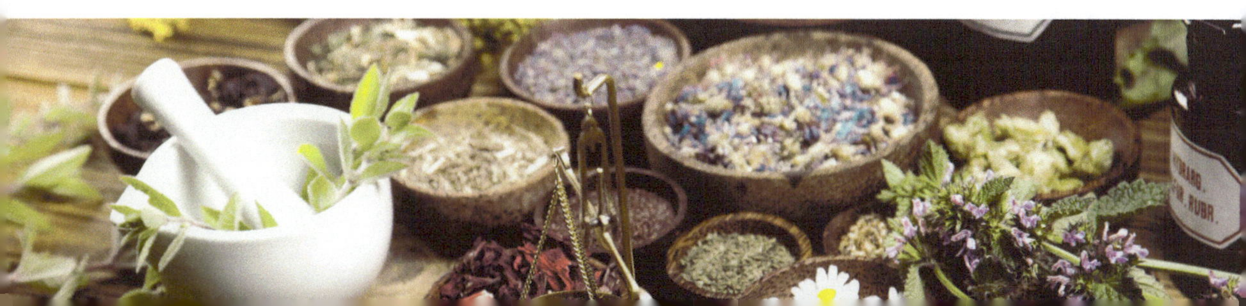

11. **TART CHERRY EXTRACT**
    Tart cherries are a natural source of melatonin and antioxidants that support healthy sleep cycles. Research suggests tart cherry juice or extract may help improve sleep duration and overall sleep quality.

12. **GLYCINE**
    Supports sleep onset and may improve sleep quality.

13. **5-HTP**
    Supports serotonin production, which plays a role in mood and sleep regulation.

14. **VITAMIN B6**
    Supports melatonin production and healthy sleep cycles.

15. **VITAMIN D3**
    Adequate vitamin D levels are associated with improved sleep regulation.

DISCLAIMER - Always consult with a qualified healthcare professional before introducing new supplements, especially if you are pregnant, nursing, or taking medication.

THE REST PRINCIPLE

You cannot heal what you never allow to rest.

Work builds strength.
Rest restores life.

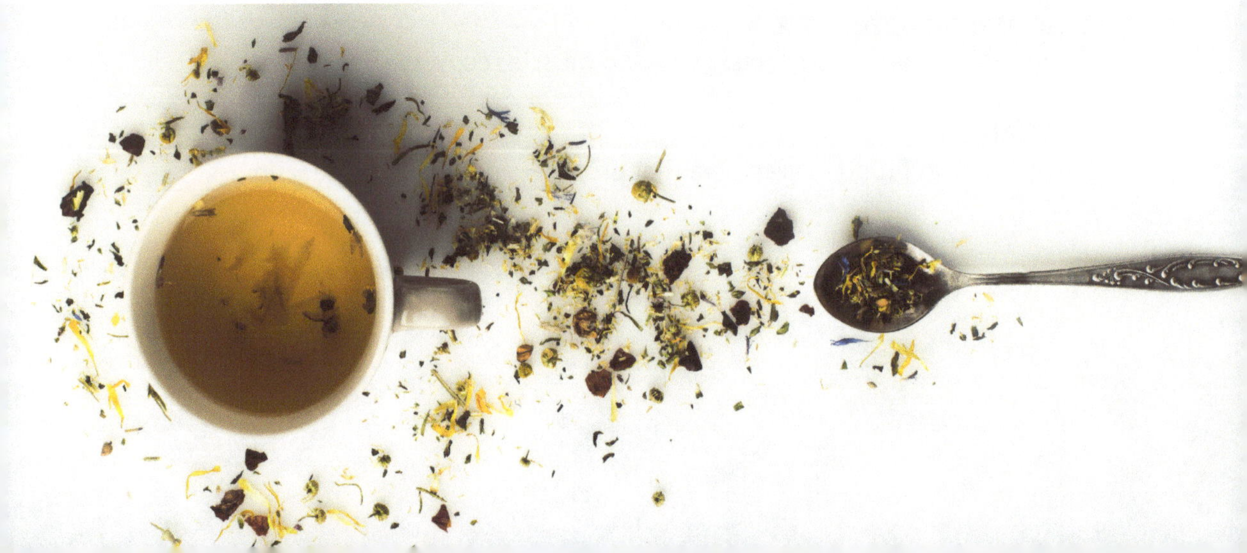

TRACKING YOUR SLEEP

Awareness leads to change. Track your sleep for one week to identify patterns affecting your rest and energy levels.

	Sunday	Monday	Tuesday	Wednesday	Thursday	Friday	Saturday
What time did you go to bed?							
How many hours did you sleep?							
How many times did you wake up?							
When did you get up?							
Did you feel rested?							
Did you have sugar cravings during the day?							

Did you drink half your body weight in ounces of water today? ______

Did you speak your daily affirmation today? ______

Did you check in with your accountability partner today? ______

(Be sure to track your sleep and other habits in your Kingdom Alliance planner.)

PILLAR 7: THE JESUS WAY

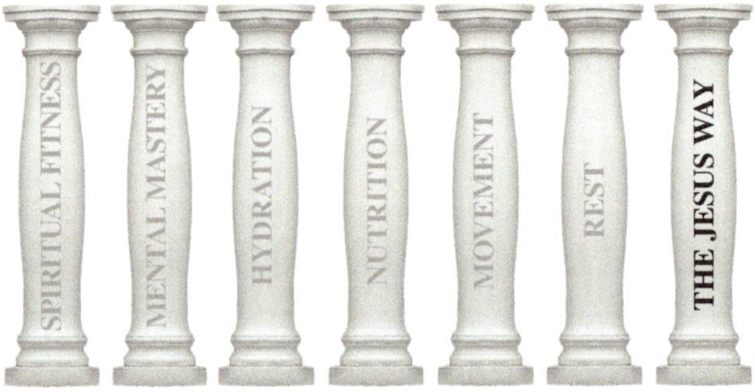

"I have come that they may have life, and have it to the full."
— John 10:10

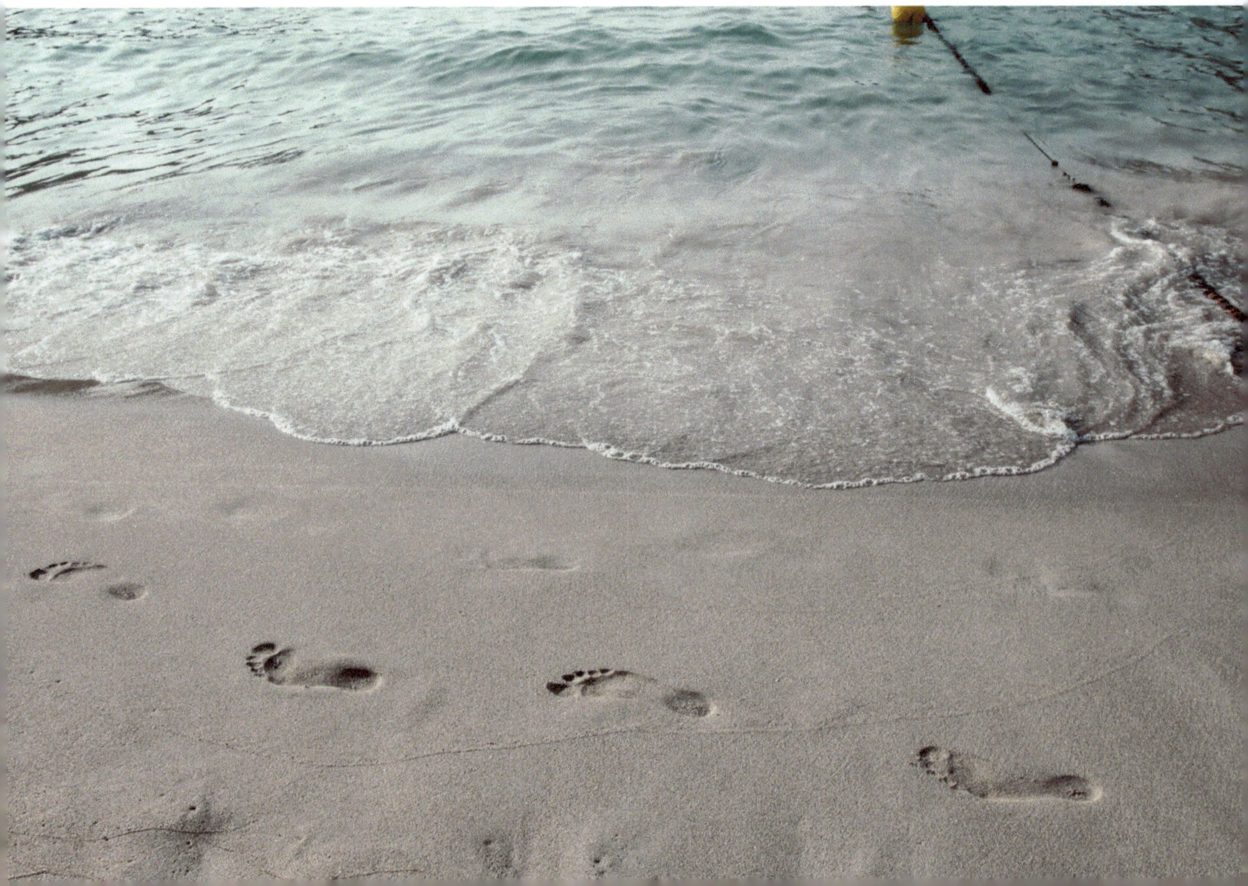

CHAPTER 15

THE JESUS WAY

God's Blueprint For Wholeness and Healing

THE SEARCH FOR A BETTER WAY

Every year, trillions of dollars are spent on pills, diets, exercise programs, and quick-fix wellness solutions. The global health and wellness industry continues to grow, yet people remain exhausted, inflamed, overweight, anxious, and confused.

Powerful industries profit from keeping people dependent on systems, products, and ongoing intervention. The loudest voices in health are often backed by money, not always by truth. And when profit drives the message, people are often left as the secondary focus, which leaves them sicker, not stronger.

That raises an important question: What if the world keeps chasing solutions that never truly solve the problem? And what if the answer was simpler, older, freer, and more powerful than we've been taught to believe?

Statistical Failure

Imagine the value of a truly proven "way" or nutritional program that worked one hundred percent of the time and helped people find their ideal weight, peak energy level, and optimal wellness without disease or sickness. And what if it was FREE?

How would that impact the world?
Who would benefit?
And what systems would crumble?

Would people embrace a truly free solution if it required surrender instead of consumption? Or would they keep trusting systems built on regulation, dependency, and man-made control?

That is the tension at the center of wellness today.

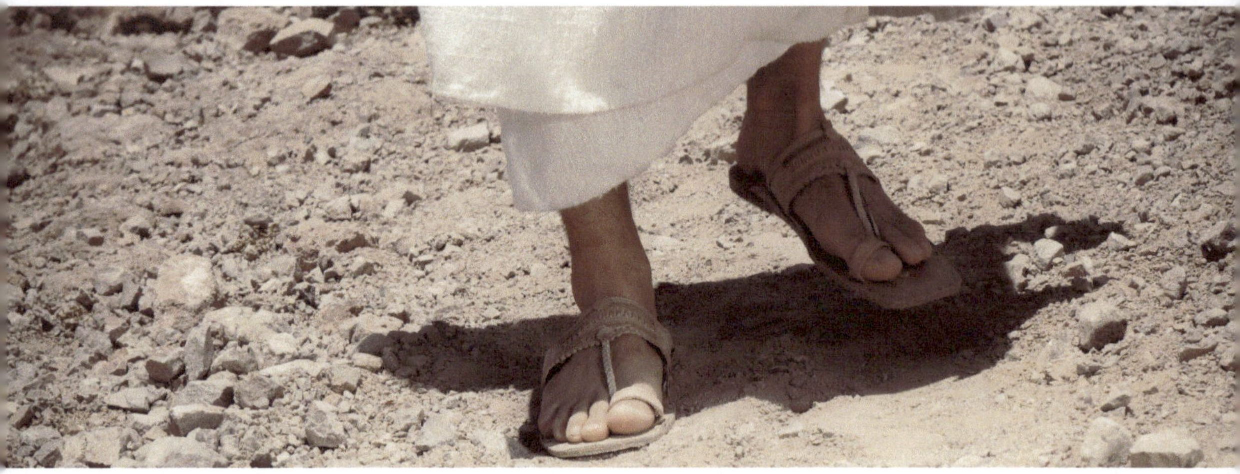

MOSAIC LAW

When we look at what happened after the fall of man, we see more than sin entering the world. We see shame, sickness, disorder, sexual immorality, worshiping of other gods, and a flood of destructive behaviors with life-threatening consequences.

From the beginning, there was a connection between human life, human choices, and the outcomes that surfaced when people chose to avoid God's commands.

In Leviticus, God gave His people detailed laws that served as an instruction manual for living in wellness, freedom, and consecration. These laws weren't to confine them but to protect them from what they didn't know.

Consider that neither science, medical education, hygiene classes, nor wellness coaching had been invented yet. God's laws had to cover every aspect of life: hygiene, food, cleansing, grooming, bodily functions, disease prevention, conflict resolution, and every detail man would encounter.

These laws were not random.

They were intentionally given in order to teach people how to live in wisdom, health, and wellness as an act of worship before a holy God.

"For I am the Lord your God. You shall therefore ***consecrate*** *yourselves, and you shall be holy; for I am holy. Neither shall you defile yourselves with any creeping thing that creeps on the earth. For I am the Lord who brings you up out of the land of Egypt, to be your God. You shall therefore be holy, for I am holy."*
— Lev. 11:44-45 (emphasis added)

Jesus Himself lived within these laws as a young child growing up in a Jewish family. He was born into a Jewish culture shaped by covenant law, consecration, and obedience.

Even Jesus obeyed the standards of the time. But the story of Scripture does not end with law.

Jesus became the law to give us freedom.

In Jesus' day, the Pharisees served as interpreters and enforcers of religious law. As this related to food and nutrition, they were the FDA (Food and Drug Administration) of the day.

Over time, layers of additional rules and traditions were added by religious leaders. What started as laws to protect mankind became rules to control mankind.

Sound familiar?

We now live in a world flooded with regulations, policies, mandates, and institutional control. There are health bills passed that contain thousands of pages detailing how a system can and will control the people, their food, and their freedoms.

The deeper problem is not merely the existence of these endless mandates, but how the human tendency is to trust those laws more than God's divine wisdom. Man-made laws have a remarkable ability to support systems that slowly replace freedom with dependency.

Yet God did not design people to live under perpetual fear, confusion, and control. He designed us to live in truth, wisdom, and Spirit-led discernment.

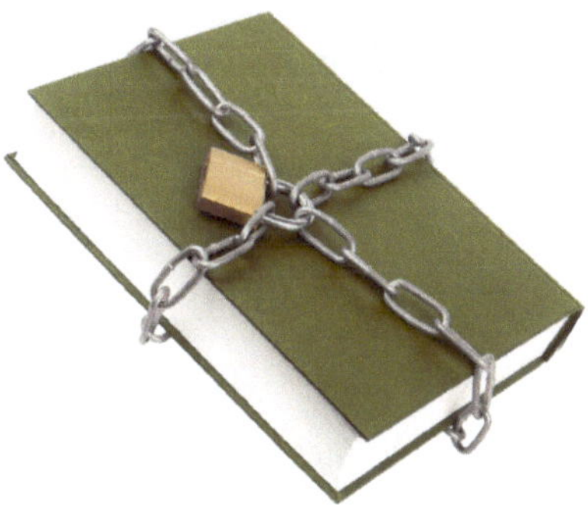

The Pharisees believed they were protecting righteousness, yet many of them had mistaken control for holiness.

Jesus refused to bow to man-made burdens masquerading as divine truth. That is one reason He was seen as dangerous. Rebellious. Unruly.

Freedom always threatens systems built on fear and manipulation.

A BETTER WAY

"For the law was given through Moses, but grace and truth (a better way) came through Jesus Christ."
— John 1:17

God knew that rules alone could never redeem humanity. No amount of regulation, sacrifice, or external compliance rules could free people from sin, fear, and death.

That is why He sent His Son.

Through Jesus' life, death, and resurrection, we are no longer justified by external rule-keeping. Food is no longer our master. Law is no longer our savior. Man-made systems no longer hold ultimate authority over the soul. Jesus became the law so we could be free.

Jesus came to show us that following a set of rules was not the path to freedom. He challenged the religious leaders of His day because they had elevated human tradition above Godly character. They focused on external defilement while neglecting inward transformation.

Jesus said:

"These people honor me with their lips, but their hearts are far from me.
They worship me in vain; their teachings are merely human rules."
- Matthew 15:8–9

Jesus did not come merely to modify behavior. He came to restore freedom, truth, and communion with the Father.

This is where everything changes. Jesus is not just a better rule.

He is the Way.

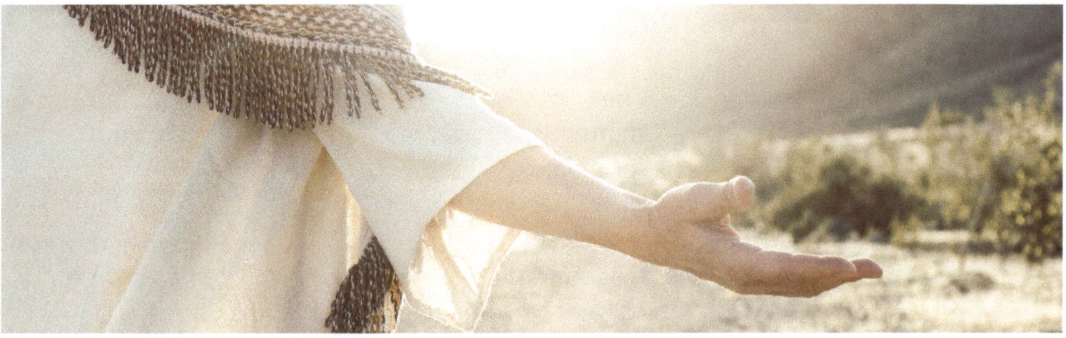

He is reaching out to show you the only lasting path out of bondage, addiction, fear, shame, and human control.

Jesus tore the veil, giving us the potential to rule and reign in dominion over sickness, disease, and the limitations of this earth. He showed us how to consecrate our food through prayer and blessing, making it a time of Holy Communion with the Father. This changed everything.

But if Jesus is the Way, then every counterfeit way must be exposed.

For generations, people have looked to rules, rituals, restrictions, and man-made systems to do what only God can do. Even in wellness, many have traded freedom for formulas and grace for food laws.

Diets may promise control, confidence, and transformation, but when they become a substitute for wisdom, surrender, and relationship with God, they lead us back into bondage. That is where the deception begins.

The Deception of DIETS

Since ancient times, food has been shaped by culture, class, pressure, image, and profit. In today's world, diets are often marketed as salvation—the answer to weight loss, energy, confidence, longevity, and health.

And while some contain practical wisdom, many become just another form of striving. Consider the endless stream of approaches that have captured public attention:

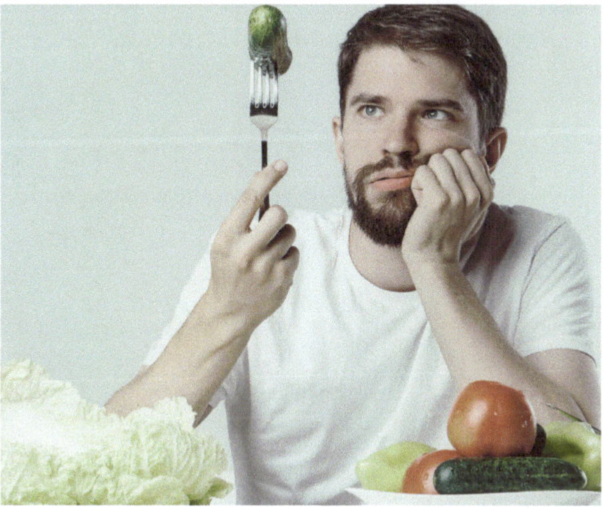

- The Cotton Ball Diet
- The Vinegar Diet
- The Cigarette Diet
- The Slimming Soap Diet
- The Tapeworm Diet
- The Low Fat Diet
- The Mediterranean Diet
- The Low Carb Diet
- The Sleeping Beauty Diet
- The Carnivore Diet
- The Keto Diet
- The Gluten-Free Diet
- The Paleo Diet

The list goes on and on and on.

Some of these offer helpful insight. But many are tied to industries that profit from confusion, identity-based eating, and the constant reinvention of food rules.

In Matthew 15, Jesus made something profoundly clear: it is not what enters a person's mouth that ultimately defiles them, but what comes out of the heart.

That does not give us permission to abuse the body with toxic foods, careless habits, or chemical overload. It means our relationship with food must be governed by wisdom, holiness, and the Holy Spirit—not fear, obsession, shame, or control.

When you study the life of Jesus, you see a higher pattern. He was never ruled by the corruption, manipulation, or monetized systems of man. He lived in honor before the Father, and He showed us how to do the same.

Freedom begins when food is no longer your master.
Freedom begins when fear is no longer your guide.
Freedom begins when grace becomes greater than the rules that once controlled you.

This is the better way.

The Gateway to ABUNDANCE & FREEDOM

If diets, rules, and man-made systems are not the answer, then where is true freedom found?

It is found in Jesus.

Jesus came to restore what sin had broken and reconnect us to the life of God. The Fall fractured more than the human heart. It disrupted creation itself. The soil was affected. The body was affected. Human appetites were affected. The harmony God designed in Eden was broken.

That means even our best efforts now take place in a fallen world.

We can pursue wisdom. We can eat cleaner. We can move our bodies. We can steward our health with honor. But no human system can fully restore what was lost through sin.

Just as good works can never save us, good habits can never make us whole apart from God.

We do not need another fad.
We do not need another food idol.
We do not need another man-made system promising salvation through self-discipline.

We need a Savior.
We need grace.
We need freedom that can only be found when we realign ourselves with God through Jesus Christ.

Food is not your savior.
Fitness is not your savior.
Supplements are not your savior.

Jesus is.

Without Him, even the best plan becomes another burden. But with Him, health becomes an overflow of covenant relationship rather than human striving.

This is the gateway to abundance and freedom.

JESUS TAUGHT SANCTIFICATION

How Jesus Redeemed the Table

Jesus knew that human appetite would be tested in many forms, including food, money, anger, lust, and the pull of self-rule. So throughout His ministry, He showed His disciples a better way to live.

Again and again, at the table and among the crowds, Jesus revealed a holy pattern. He did not approach food casually or consume without awareness. He received it, blessed it, broke it, and shared it. In doing so, He showed us that nourishment was never meant to be merely physical. It was meant to be consecrated.

No matter what food, bread, or drink is placed before you, Jesus modeled a pattern that can bring intention, gratitude, and holiness back into the act of eating:

1. Receive it (Authority)
2. Bless it (Gratitude and Honor)
3. Break it (Remembrance)
4. Share it (Generosity)

"And He took bread, gave thanks and broke it, and gave it to them, saying, 'This is My body given for you; do this in remembrance of Me.'"
— Luke 22:19

"Now it came to pass, as He sat at the table with them, that He took bread, blessed and broke it, and gave it to them."
— Luke 24:30

"Then He commanded the multitudes to sit down on the grass. And He took the five loaves and the two fish, and looking up to heaven, He blessed and broke and gave the loaves to the disciples; and the disciples gave to the multitudes."
— Matthew 14:19

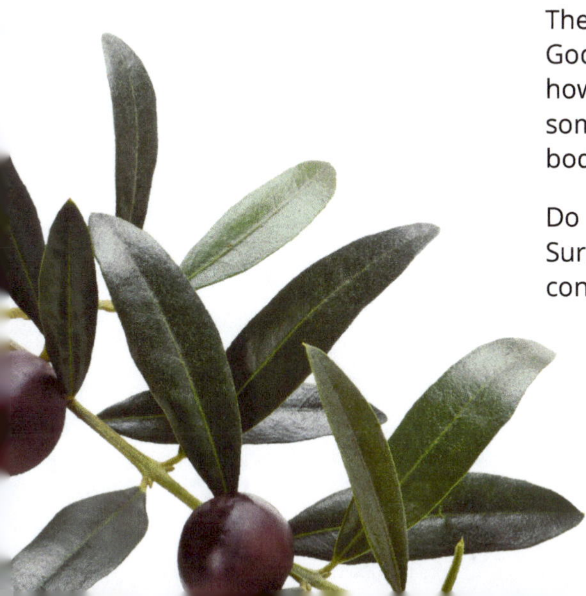

The greatest path to wellness is wisdom, allowing God to teach you what to eat, drink, think, and how to live. But beyond choosing the right food is something deeper: sanctifying what enters your body through prayer.

Do what Jesus did. Receive it with gratitude. Surrender it to God. Honor Him in the way you consume it.

This is the better way.

This is freedom.

This is how Jesus redeemed the table.

CHAPTER 16

THE JESUS WAY OF RENEWAL

God's Design for Total Wellness

SPIRITUAL FASTING

The Divine Reset for Body, Mind, and Spirit

Fasting is not about deprivation. It is about divine alignment. It is not merely about what you give up, but about what God restores in you as you make room for Him.

From Genesis to Jesus, fasting has been a pathway to clarity, consecration, and deeper communion with God. It is both a spiritual discipline and a divine strategy for renewal. When we quiet the cravings of the flesh and yield our appetites to the Spirit, our hearts become more attentive to God and our bodies begin to respond to His design.

Fasting is a Key to Kingdom Renewal
God designed the body with rhythms of rest, repair, and restoration. Fasting works with those rhythms. It creates an intentional pause that allows the body to reset while the spirit becomes more sensitive to the voice of God.

Your Body's Built-In Cleansing System
Science is now confirming what Scripture has revealed for generations: fasting activates healing and repair processes in the body. One of the most remarkable is "autophagy," the body's built-in recycling system, in which damaged cellular material is cleared out so healthier cells can function more efficiently.

A Kingdom Reset for Hormones and Metabolism
Fasting can also support mental clarity, insulin sensitivity, and hormonal balance. It has been associated with increased production of BDNF, a protein linked to brain health. It helps calm internal noise, sharpen focus, and bring the body back under order while bringing the heart back into surrender.

Fasting is a gift from God, designed to ensure that your body remains a clean, pure, and powerful temple of the Holy Spirit.

"Do you not know that your bodies are temples of the Holy Spirit, who is in you?"
— 1 Corinthians 6:19

WHEN THE BODY BEGINS TO RESET

When the body is given space to rest, reset, and recover, some of its most powerful healing processes begin to awaken.

Inflammation, Be Silenced

Inflammation is one of the hidden drivers behind many chronic conditions. Fasting may help reduce inflammatory stress in the body, creating space for greater balance, healing, and clarity.

Spiritually, fasting quiets internal noise. Physically, it gives the body room to recalibrate.

The Sabbath of Your Gut

Even your digestive system needs rest. Constant eating keeps the gut working without pause. Fasting gives it a break—a chance to recover, reduce bloating, support immunity, and restore internal balance.

Sometimes, one of the most healing things you can do is stop overworking the systems God designed to serve you.

A Divine Reboot

Research continues to show that extended fasting can trigger profound metabolic shifts. As the body moves into deeper ketosis, it begins using stored fat for fuel, improving insulin sensitivity, reducing chronic inflammation, and activating autophagy, the body's built-in cellular cleanup process. For many people, this leads to clearer thinking, greater energy, metabolic reset, and renewed resilience.

The Bread of Life

Fasting reminds us that food is not our deepest source. God is.

When Jesus said, "Man shall not live by bread alone, but by every word that proceeds from the mouth of God," (Matthew 4:4), He revealed a deeper truth: the human soul was never meant to live on physical nourishment alone.

Fasting reorders desire. It teaches the body to be still and the spirit to hunger for what truly satisfies.

Vitality and Renewal

Research continues to explore how fasting may support cellular resilience, metabolic flexibility, and healthy aging. But beyond the science, fasting builds discipline, dependence on God, and spiritual sensitivity.

As we empty ourselves before Him, we make room for renewal in body, mind, and spirit.

STAYING GROUNDED

Reconnecting With the Earth God Made

From the beginning, God designed humanity to live in relationship with creation. The earth was not given merely as scenery, but as provision, rhythm, and place.

We were made to live close to what God made.

"Then the Lord God formed man from the dust of the ground and breathed into his nostrils the breath of life."
— Genesis 2:7

Modern life has pulled many people away from those rhythms. We spend our days indoors, surrounded by artificial light, synthetic environments, screens, stress, and constant stimulation. But the body often responds with peace when we return to the simplicity of creation.

Standing barefoot on grass, soil, sand, or stone can become more than a pleasant habit. It can be a quiet act of reconnection and a way to slow down, calm the nervous system, and remember where we came from.

Some call this "grounding." But long before it became a wellness term, Scripture revealed that creation itself carries the wisdom, order, and goodness of God.

The heavens declare the glory of God; the skies proclaim the work of His hands."
— Psalm 19:1

When we step outside, walk near the water, feel the grass beneath our feet, or sit quietly under the open sky, something begins to settle. The soul becomes quieter. The body becomes less hurried. The mind becomes more attentive.

This is not about worshipping nature. It is about returning to the created order God called good. Take off your shoes. Feel the earth. Sit in the sun. Walk near the water. Return often to the quiet places where creation still testifies of God's goodness.

Sometimes, one of the most healing things you can do is step away from the artificial world and place your body back in contact with the earth God made.

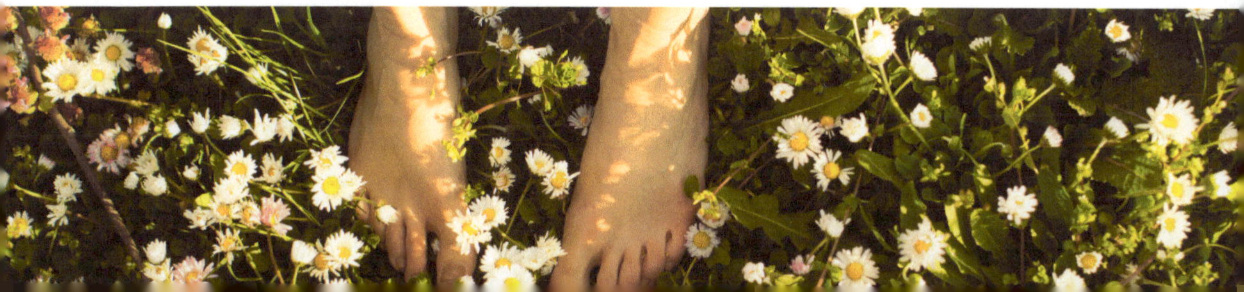

THE HEALING RHYTHM OF LIGHT

4 Ways Light Shapes Your Health

From the beginning, God designed light as a carrier of order, rhythm, and life. The sun is not merely decorative. It signals wakefulness, supports biological timing, and helps regulate the body's natural cycles of energy, hormones, digestion, and rest.

"And God said, 'Let there be light,' and there was light."
— Genesis 1:3

Scientists call it the circadian rhythm, regulated by the suprachiasmatic nucleus, which is just a very sophisticated way of saying God built your body to respond to light.

1. **Light Sets Your Internal Clock**
   Your circadian rhythm is the body's built-in 24-hour clock. It regulates sleep, hormone release, digestion, body temperature, energy, and alertness. God designed your body to respond to light cues—waking you in the morning and preparing you for rest at night.

   Simple Takeaway:
   Your body is always listening to light.

2. **Morning Light Signals Life**
   When morning light enters the eyes, it tells the brain it is time to wake up. This boosts alertness, supports serotonin production, and helps set the body up for healthier melatonin release later that evening.

   Just ten to twenty minutes of morning sunlight can support:
   - better sleep
   - improved mood
   - sharper focus
   - healthier energy rhythms

   Simple Takeaway:
   Morning light helps set your body's clock.

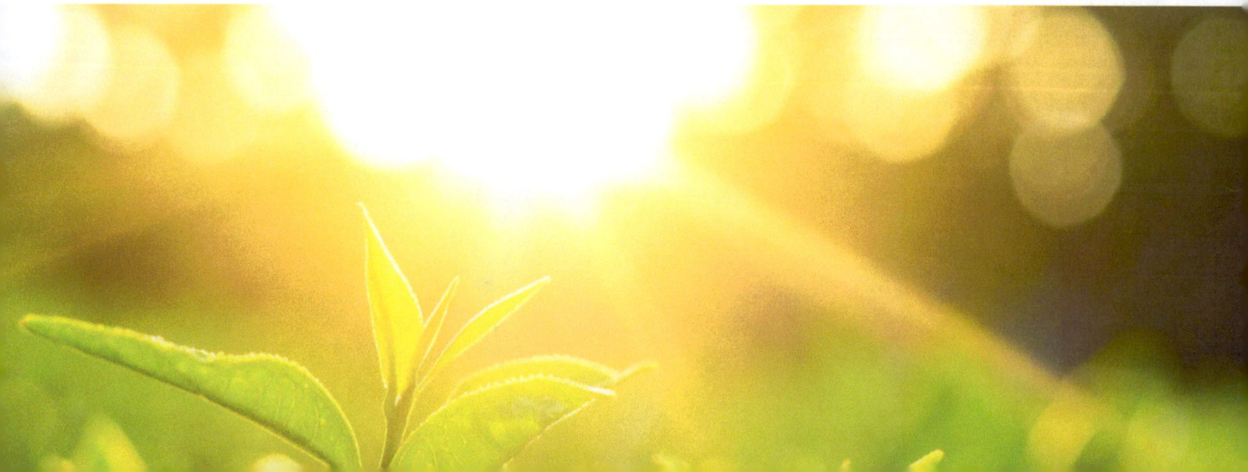

3. **Blue Light Disrupts the Rhythm**

   Not all light helps the body equally. Blue light from phones, tablets, TVs, and computers can confuse your internal clock—especially at night. Instead of signaling rest, it tells the brain to stay awake, making it harder to wind down and release melatonin.

   Too much blue light exposure may contribute to:
   - trouble falling asleep
   - poor sleep quality
   - increased stress
   - eye fatigue
   - circadian disruption

   Simple Takeaway:
   What the sun helps restore, screens can easily disrupt.

4. **God Designed Light to Heal**

   God created light before He created man. Light is woven into the order of creation. It is part of the rhythm of waking, working, repairing, and resting. Jesus also lived in harmony with the day. He rose early, withdrew to pray, and moved in oneness with God and His creation.

   "Very early in the morning, while it was still dark, Jesus got up, left the house, and went off to a solitary place, where He prayed."
   — Mark 1:35

   And beyond physical light, Jesus revealed the deeper truth:

   "I am the light of the world. Whoever follows Me will never walk in darkness, but will have the light of life."
   — John 8:12

   The sun can awaken the body.
   But Jesus awakens the soul.

   Simple Takeaway:
   Light is one of God's greatest gifts for the body's restoration.

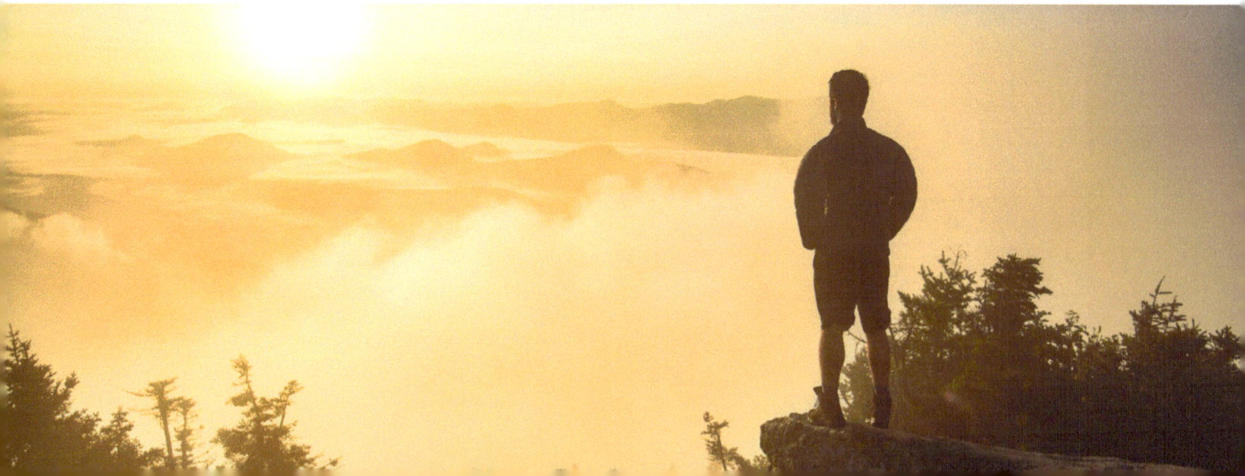

CHAPTER 17
RISE, REBUILD, RULE, AND REIGN

Rooted to Flourish in Every Season

On the island of Crete, in the village of Ano Vouves, stands an ancient olive tree widely considered one of the oldest in the world. Some estimates place it at more than 2,000 years old. Others suggest it could be far older. No one can say with certainty exactly how old it is. But one thing is certain:

It is still alive.
It is still standing.
It is still bearing fruit.

Think about that.

Empires have risen and fallen.
Governments have come and gone.
Wars have been fought.
Generations have lived and died.
And that tree is still there.

Standing.
Rooted.
Weathered.
Scarred.
Beaten.
Treasured

And through
it all...

**That sacred
olive tree
is still
bearing fruit.**

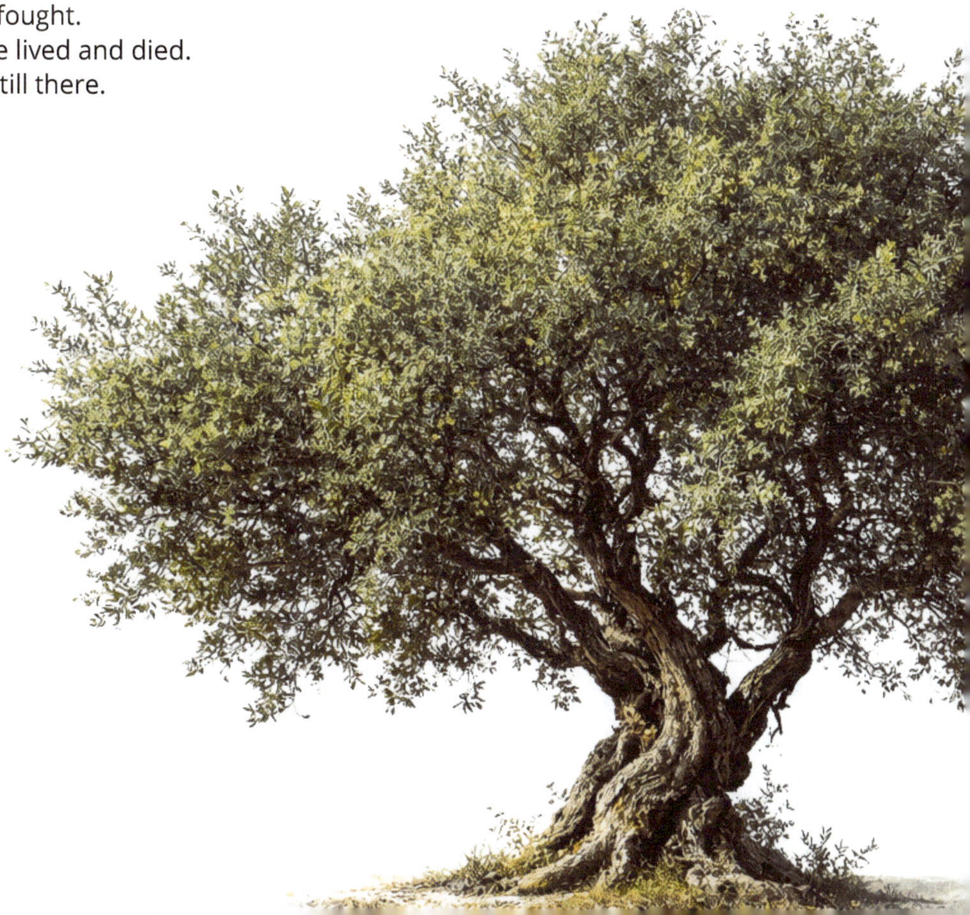

Its trunk is twisted and hollowed with age. Its form is marked by time and pressure. Yet it still produces olives. And in one of the most poetic details of all, branches from that ancient tree were used to weave wreaths for Olympic victors, connecting endurance with victory, age with honor, and rootedness with reward.

That is a picture of the life God wants to build in you.

Not a rushed life.
Not a shallow life.
Not a flashy life that burns bright for a moment and then collapses.

But a rooted life.
A fruitful life.
A consecrated life.
A life that can withstand pressure without losing peace.

The olive tree does not become strong overnight. It grows slowly. Quietly. Deeply.

Long before fruit appears on its branches, something far more important is happening beneath the surface. Its roots are stretching downward, anchoring, reaching, and drawing from hidden places. While other trees may grow fast and look impressive for a season, the olive tree is built for endurance. It can withstand heat, drought, wind, and pressure because its strength is not based on speed. It is based on depth.

And maybe that is where you are today.

Pressed.
Pruned.
Weathered.
Tired.

But you are not abandoned.

Because in the Kingdom, pressing is never pointless. It is powerful, full of purpose, and a necessary ingredient to endurance.

Sometimes the very seasons that felt like they were crushing you were the seasons God was using to deepen your roots. Through every hardship, every holy interruption, every act of surrender, every hidden prayer, and every small act of obedience, He has been doing deeper work than you could see.

Roots matter.

Because when your life is rooted in God's wisdom, you can withstand what once took you out. You can live with peace where there used to be panic. You can live with discipline where there used to be chaos. You can live with strength where there used to be depletion. You can live with clarity where there used to be confusion.

You were never meant to live like a withering branch, disconnected from the source. **You were made to flourish.**

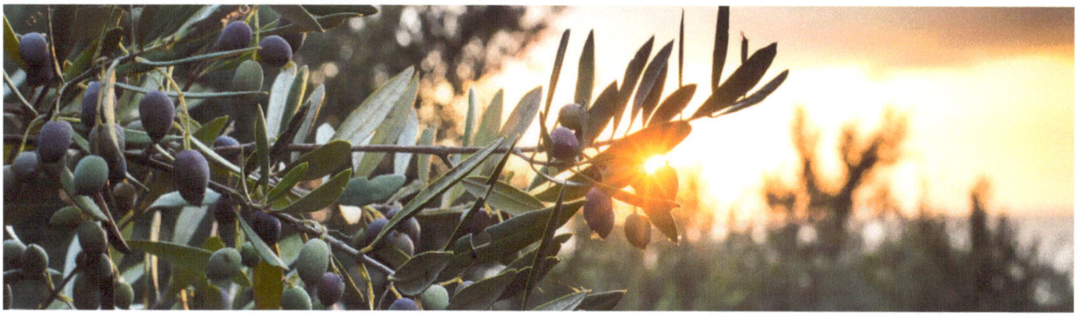

The Life God Designed

From the very beginning, God's design for humanity was wholeness.

He formed man from the dust of the earth, breathed life into him, and placed him in a garden filled with beauty, order, nourishment, and peace. There was no striving there. No confusion. No addiction. No burnout. No sickness. No fractured identity. Humanity lived in rhythm with God, in harmony with creation, and in full dependence on Heaven.

But the fall fractured more than a relationship. It disrupted the whole ecosystem of human flourishing.

It affected the ground.
It affected the body.
It affected the mind.
It affected appetites, desires, work, rest, and identity.

Since then, mankind has been trying to rebuild by effort what can only be restored by alignment.

That is why this book is not just about health.
It is about returning.

Returning to God's wisdom.
Returning to His order.
Returning to the rhythms that restore.
Returning to the life Heaven intended.

THE SEVEN PILLARS IN REVIEW

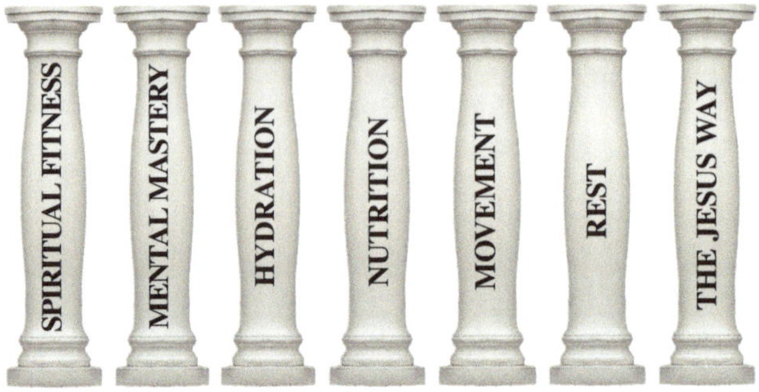

You have walked through the seven pillars of optimal wellness, but in truth, they are more than pillars. They are your scaffolding for life. They are invitations into right alignment with God. They are practical ways to steward the body, mind, and spirit He entrusted to you.

If you will let them, they will lead you back to a life that is rooted, resilient, and Fueled by God's design.

Spiritual Fitness reminds you that real health begins in the spirit. Your body may be the vessel, but your spirit is the source of your direction, discernment, and strength.

Mental Mastery calls you to renew your mind, because the life you build is shaped by the thoughts you believe. Peace, clarity, and resilience all begin with what you allow to rule your inner world.

Hydration teaches you to honor the most basic gift of physical life: water. It is a daily reminder that your body needs replenishment, and so does your soul.

Nutrition calls you back to wisdom, simplicity, and true nourishment. It invites you to stop consuming what depletes you and honor your body with what was designed to sustain you.

Movement reminds you that the body was made to move, strengthen, work, and engage. Now you can move it with intention to heal and restore what you've lost.

Rest teaches you that pausing is not weakness. It is wisdom. Sleep, stillness, gratitude, laughter, peace, and Sabbath are all part of Heaven's answer to a world addicted to hurry.

The Jesus Way reveals the deepest truth of all: no habit, plan, supplement, or strategy can take the place of surrender. True wholeness is not found in a formula. It is found in a Person.

These pillars are the scaffolding you need to bring freedom, wholeness, and healing to your life.

At this point, you may be tempted to turn these pages into a checklist.

Drink more water.
Sleep more.
Eat cleaner.
Move daily.
Pray more.
Think better.
Fast consistently.

And yes, those actions matter.

But this book was never meant to become another stack of rules sitting on your shoulders.

**This is not behavior modification for the sake of appearance.
This is transformation for the sake of Kingdom alignment.**

No supplement on earth can give you peace.
No diet can heal your soul.
No workout can restore your identity.
No routine can replace surrender.
No amount of information can produce revelation.

You do not need another trend.
You need truth.
You need grace.
You need wisdom that changes not only
your habits, but your hunger.

**That is why this book does not end
with a plan. It ends with a call.**

A call to live differently.
A call to think differently.
A call to steward your body as a temple
and your life as an offering.
A call to stop surviving and start abiding.

**Real change happens when your life comes
back under the Lordship of Jesus Christ.**

That is where healing deepens.
That is where peace returns.
That is where clarity sharpens.
That is where discipline stops
feeling like punishment and
starts becoming worship.

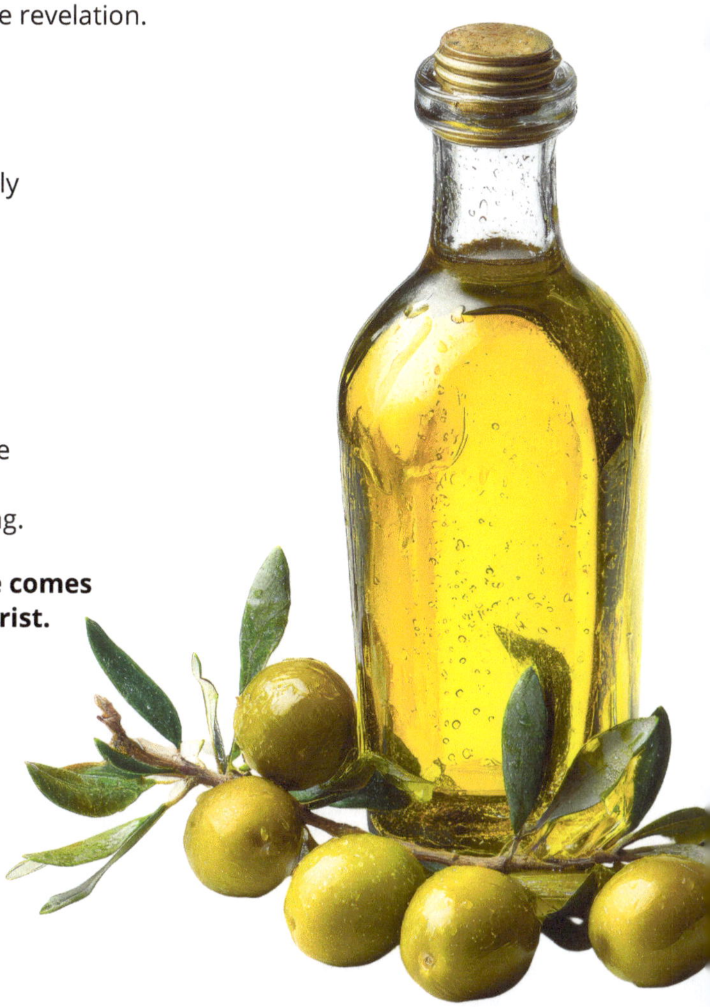

RISE, REBUILD, RULE, AND REIGN

Rise

Rise out of passivity.
Rise out of confusion.
Rise out of addiction to the patterns that held you back.
Rise out of the lie that says this is just how life has to be.
Rise in your thinking.
Rise in your standards.
Rise in your stewardship.
Rise in your expectation.

You are not called to drift through life with symptoms and settle for survival. You are called to wake up, live with intention, steward your body, and rise into a life of purpose.

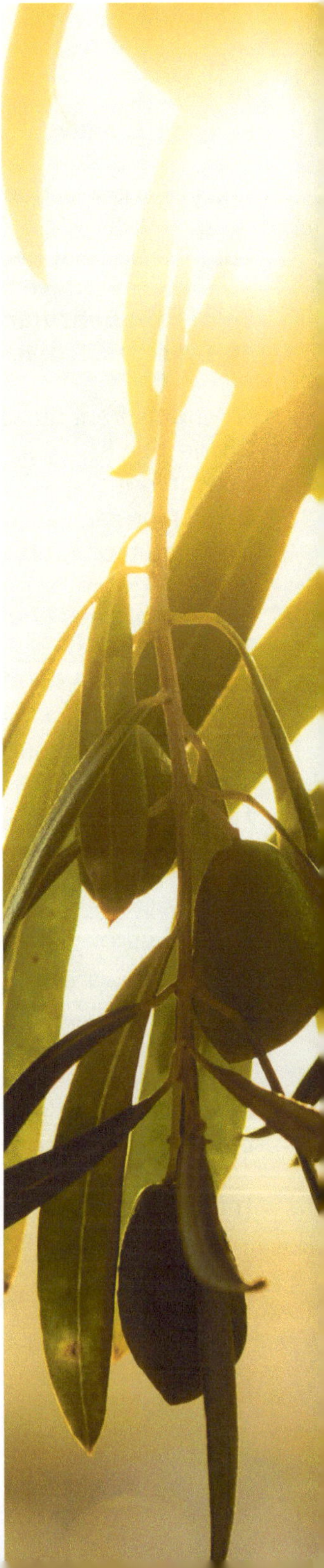

Rebuild

Some readers will need to build for the first time. Others will need to rebuild what has been neglected, misused, or broken down over time.

Rebuild your spirit with daily communion with God.
Rebuild your mind with truth.
Rebuild your body with rest, water, nourishment, and movement.
Rebuild your schedule with margin.
Rebuild your home with peace.
Rebuild your appetite with healthy choices.
Rebuild your life with godly disciplines.

Olive trees might grow slowly, but they endure when others fall.

The life that lasts is rarely built in a rush.

Small acts of obedience, practiced daily with consistency, become a life of strength over time.

A glass of water.
A walk in the sun.
A better choice at lunch.
A simple fast.
Ten minutes in prayer.
A screen turned off at night.
A firm "no" to the flesh.
A surrendered "yes" to God.
This is how rebuilding begins.

PART THREE:
GROW

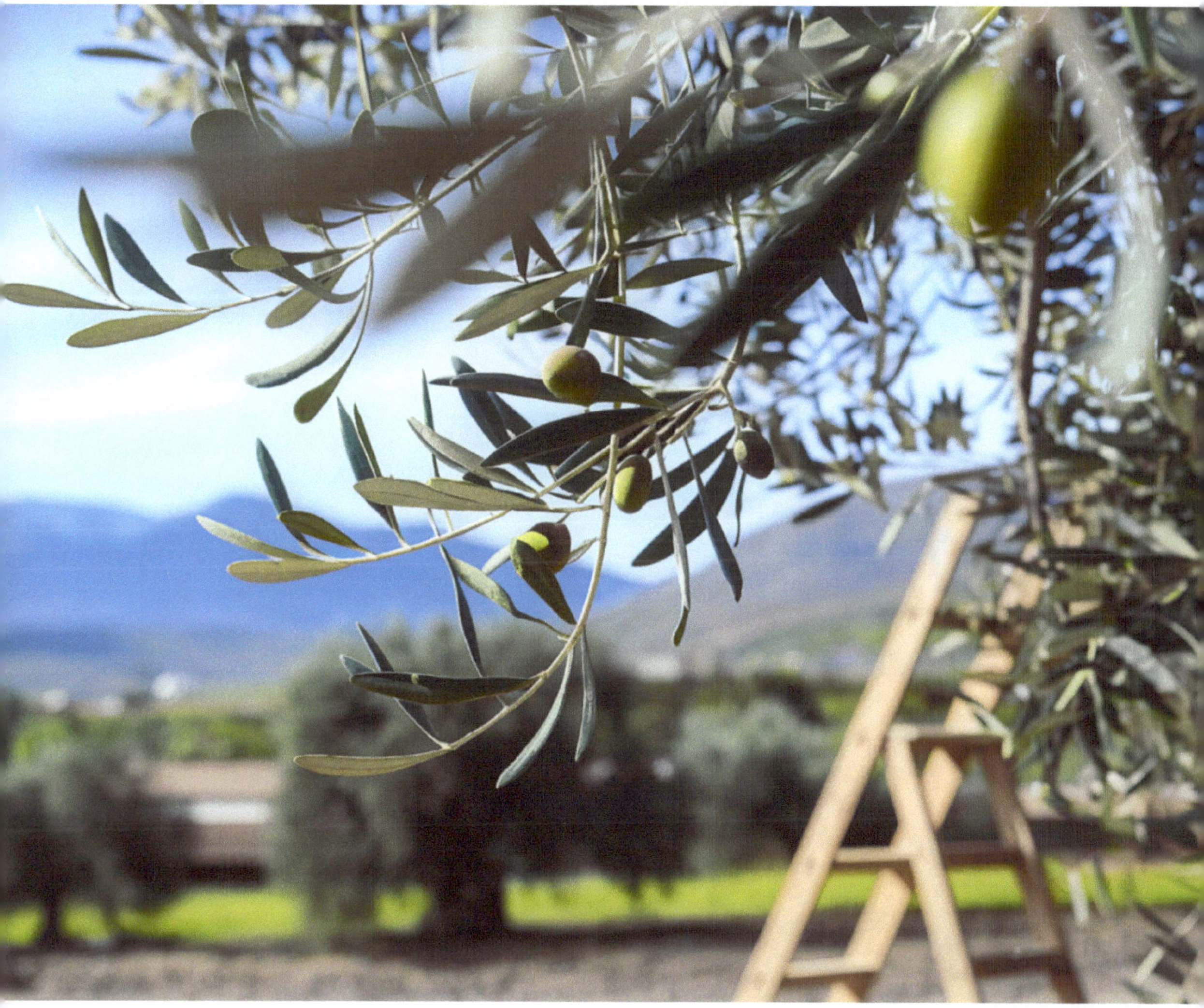

"His branches shall spread, and his beauty shall be as the olive tree, and his smell as Lebanon."

– Hosea 14:6

THE 7X CHALLENGE

7 Days. 7 Weeks. Total Realignment.

You were not created to live exhausted, inflamed, distracted, overfed, and spiritually disconnected. You were created to live awake, clear, disciplined, and fully aligned with God's design for your life. That is what this challenge is about.

The Fueled 7X Challenge is a forty-nine-day journey of intentional wellness, spiritual focus, and practical obedience. Over the next seven weeks, you will begin strengthening Kingdom-aligned disciplines that help you cleanse your body, reset your appetite, renew your mind, and draw closer to God.

This is not just about losing weight.

It is about losing what has been weighing you down.
It is about breaking cycles.
Restoring discipline.
Choosing life.
And learning to glorify God with your body in a fresh, intentional way.

Each week will give you practical tools to help you move forward with wisdom and consistency. Some days will challenge your habits. Some will expose your cravings. Some will strengthen your resolve. But all of it is designed to help you live with greater freedom, clarity, and self-control.

You do not need to do this perfectly. You simply need to do it willingly and consistently. This is not a performance-driven discipline. It is a surrendered, relationship-driven realignment with God.

As you move through this challenge, you will learn how fasting, detox, nourishment, movement, prayer, and intentional choices can work together to support both physical healing and spiritual renewal.

Later in this section, we will also look at the example of Daniel, who chose conviction over compromise, reminding us that what we consume shapes who we become.

LET'S PRAY

Father God, thank You for the honor of living as a temple and carrier of Your Spirit. Forgive me for any way I have neglected to treat my body with the holiness, honor, and excellence it deserves. Realign my thoughts, choices, and desires with Your best for my life. Give me the strength to finish strong and the discipline to complete this challenge with excellence. In Jesus' name, amen.

According to many health experts, it takes time for the body to reset old patterns and establish new ones. That is one reason this challenge is built around forty-nine days—seven days a week for seven weeks of intentional change.

But this is about more than habit formation.

The Fueled 7X Challenge is a practical and spiritual journey designed to help you cleanse your body, renew your mind, strengthen your discipline, and deepen your connection with God. Over the next seven weeks, you will begin replacing survival habits with life-giving rhythms that support wholeness from the inside out.

Each week, you will focus on simple but intentional actions that support your health and your spiritual alignment. These may include fasting, hydration, food choices, movement, rest, prayer, and reflection. Some changes will feel small. Others may stretch you. But every step is designed to move you toward greater clarity, energy, peace, and self-control.

This challenge is not about perfection.
It is about pursuing purpose and alignment.
It is not about punishing your body.
It is about honoring it as the Temple of the Holy Spirit.
It is not about chasing quick results or the latest fads.
It is about building sustainable disciplines that help you live stronger, think more clearly, and walk more closely with God.

You may experience physical transformation during these forty-nine days. Many people do. But the greatest transformation is often deeper than the scale. It shows up in your discipline, your focus, your mood, your cravings, your confidence, and your spiritual sensitivity.

This is your invitation to begin again.
To reset what has been out of order.
To release what has been weighing you down.
And to rebuild from a place of wisdom, grace, and intentional obedience.

BEFORE YOU BEGIN

Take your "before" photo, complete your personal assessment, and set aside time to pray over these next forty-nine days. Ask God to guide you, strengthen you, and reveal what He wants to heal, reset, and restore.

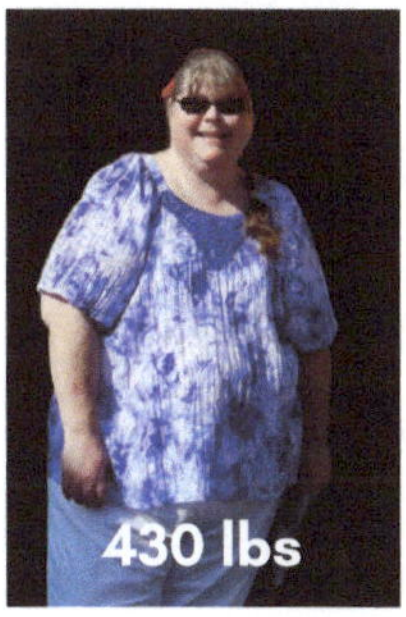

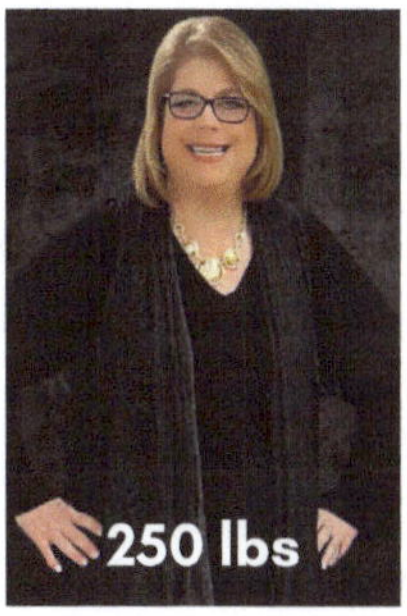

THE 7X CHALLENGE

7 Days. 7 Weeks. Total Realignment.

NUTRITION

FOOD IS FUEL FOR LIFE

Over the next seven weeks, your food choices will become more intentional, nourishing, and aligned with the way God designed your body to function. The acronym F.O.O.D. will help you stay on track and focused on what matters most.

F

WEEK 1: FREE YOURSELF

Remove processed, man-made junk foods, including sugary drinks, fried foods, alcohol, and heavily processed snacks.

O

WEEK 2: ORGANIC UPGRADE

Choose the cleanest foods available to you, focusing on vegetables, quality proteins, and fruit in moderation.

O

WEEK 3: OBSERVE THE PLATE PROTOCOL

Build your meals using this simple pattern:

50% above-ground vegetables
25% protein: meat, fish, eggs, cheese, or nuts
25% root vegetables, legumes, or other whole-food carbohydrates

D

WEEKS 4–6: DANIEL FAST

Complete a Daniel Fast, ending with a 3-day water fast if appropriate for your health and experience level.

Important note: If you have a diagnosed medical condition, are pregnant, nursing, taking medication, or have any health concerns, consult your doctor first. If needed, complete a modified version using raw vegetables, limited fruit, or another wise adjustment.

WEEK 7: RETURN TO THE FUELED FOR LIFE PLATE

Return to the Fueled for Life Plate Protocol in Chapter 10 and consider making it your long-term foundation for daily living.

Simple Reminder:

Food is not your savior. But it can become either a burden or a blessing, depending on what you choose.

Meat and dairy should be organic, pasture-raised or grass-fed, which will avoid the antibiotics, growth hormones, pesticides, and herbicides used in conventional farming. Fish should be wild caught, and if canned, avoid the ones in any oils other than extra virgin olive oil.

THE 7X CHALLENGE

7 Days. 7 Weeks. Total Realignment.

REST

RESTORATION AND RENEWAL

Your body heals when it rests. During this challenge, protect your evenings and make room for restoration. Sleep is not laziness. It is obedience to the way God designed your body to recover, reset, and renew.

R

RELEASE THE DAY

- Do not carry the weight of the day into the night. Let go of pressure, unfinished tasks, and mental clutter.

E

ELIMINATE EVENING STIMULATION

- Turn off electronics, dim the lights, and reduce unnecessary noise and input by 9:00 p.m.

S

SETTLE YOUR SOUL

- Create a simple evening routine that helps your body and mind slow down. Breathe, reflect, read Scripture, or sit quietly with God.

T

TRUST GOD WHILE YOU SLEEP

- Aim for at least 7–8 hours of sleep, trusting that God restores what striving cannot.

"In peace I will lie down and sleep, for You alone, Lord, make me dwell in safety."
— Psalm 4:8

THE 7X CHALLENGE

7 Days. 7 Weeks. Total Realignment.

MOVEMENT

STRENGTH FOR THE JOURNEY

Your body was created to move. During this challenge, exercise is not punishment. It is stewardship. Movement helps increase energy, support detoxification, build strength, and bring your body back into alignment with God's design.

M

MOVE DAILY

- Aim for at least 30 minutes of intentional movement, 5 days a week.

O

OPERATE IN YOUR FAT BURNING ZONE

- Spend 15–30 minutes in your Fat Burning Zone to build endurance and maximize fuel efficiency.

V

VALUE STRENGTH TRAINING

- Spend 15–30 minutes strengthening your body through weights, resistance bands, bodyweight exercises, or other functional movement.

E

ELEVATE THROUGH WORSHIP

- Praise and worship while you move. Thank God for strength, healing, and breath. Let movement become part of your communion with Him.

"For in Him we live and move and have our being."
— Acts 17:28

THE 7X CHALLENGE

7 Days. 7 Weeks. Total Realignment.

THE JESUS WAY

P.R.A.Y. OVER IT ALL

Jesus never lived rushed, reactive, or ruled by the flesh. He lived surrendered, attentive, and led by the Father. That is the invitation of this challenge. Not simply to eat better or become more disciplined, but to let every decision become an act of communion with God. The Jesus Way begins by slowing down long enough to listen. Before you move, respond, or consume, you pray.

P

PAUSE

- Give thanks before you eat and honor God as the source of your blessings.

R

REFLECT

- Reflect God daily by being a living conduit of His character.

"The fruit of the Spirit is love, joy, peace, patience, kindness, goodness, faithfulness, gentleness, self-control… "
— Galatians 5:22-23

A

ASK

- Ask God to bless your food and multiply it as nutrition to your body. When you fast, ask God how you can serve Him best in your time of sacrifice.

Y

YIELD

- Surrender the impulse to overeat or be driven by addictions or emotions. Let your obedience become an act of worship.

"Always be joyful. Never stop praying. Be thankful in all circumstances, for this is God's will for you who belong to Christ Jesus."
— 1 Thessalonians 5:16-18

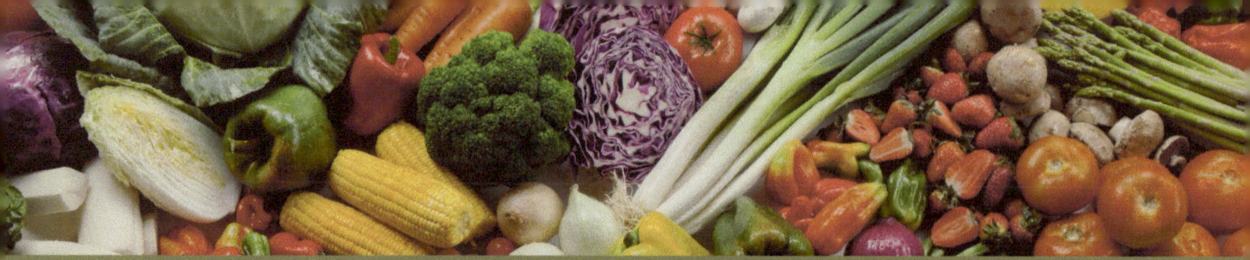

THE POWER OF F.O.O.D. FASTING

The ***Fueled 7X Challenge*** is so much more than a fitness or nutritional challenge. It is about creating space for God to reset your body, renew your mind, and realign your habits.

Fasting is one of the most powerful ways to break unhealthy cycles, quiet the noise of the flesh, and restore clarity. It teaches you how to say no to what has been ruling you so you can say yes to what gives you life.

Throughout this challenge, you will use the F.O.O.D. framework to make simple, intentional choices with what you eat. Over the next seven weeks, you will progressively remove what burdens the body, strengthen what nourishes it, and create healthier habits that make room for deeper communion with God.

This challenge includes:
A season of food awareness and intentional eating.
A return to whole, living foods.
The Fueled for Life Plate Protocol.
A focused Daniel Fast.
A final water fast for those who are able and medically cleared.

The goal is freedom.

Daniel modeled this kind of conviction when he chose restraint over compromise and trusted God with the outcome. His decision did not weaken him. It strengthened him. That is the invitation here, too.

As you begin, remember this: fasting is not just about what you are giving up. It is about what you are making room for.

"When you fast..."
— Matthew 6:16

"'Please test your servants for ten days: Give us nothing but vegetables to eat and water to drink. Then compare our appearance with that of the young men who eat the royal food, and treat your servants in accordance with what you see.' So he agreed to this and tested them for ten days. At the end of the ten days they looked healthier and better nourished than any of the young men who ate the royal food."
— Daniel 1:12 -15

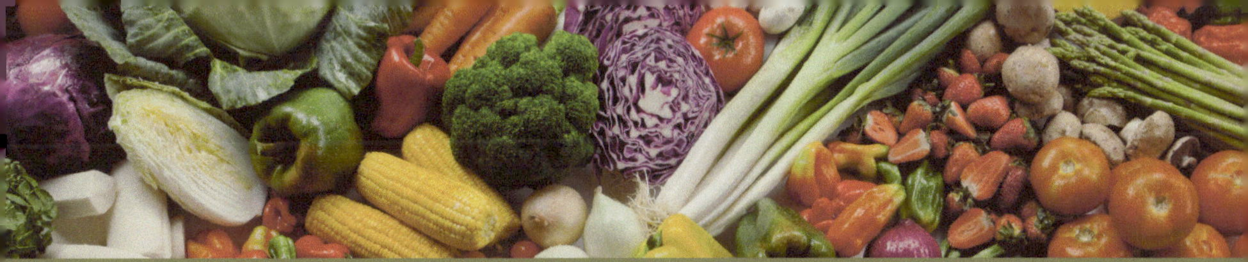

THE POWER OF F.O.O.D. FASTING

When God calls us to fast, He is not trying to deprive us. He is teaching us how to live led by the Spirit instead of ruled by cravings, appetites, and impulses. Fasting is one of the clearest ways to bring the flesh back into proper order.

"So I say, walk by the Spirit, and you will not gratify the desires of the flesh."
— Galatians 5:16

"The flesh" includes our feelings, desires, thoughts, cravings, addictions, and our poor dietary choices. When we fast, we tell our flesh that it DOES NOT rule us. Our body must stop demanding and start listening.

That is why fasting strengthens not only your discipline, but your discernment. As the noise of the flesh quiets down, the voice of God becomes easier to recognize.

It's like having a GPS system that suddenly comes online and guides you in the way you should go. Without GPS, your journey may take twice as long because you get lost along the way.

The Holy Spirit is your Heavenly GPS, guiding you in the way you should go.

While the main benefit of fasting is intimacy with the Father, God also knew that fasting was a key component to living in divine health because it gives your body a sacred pause. It allows your digestive system to rest, supports healthier insulin levels, and helps your body shift into repair mode.

Research continues to show that fasting can support weight loss, reduce inflammation, improve metabolic health, and activate autophagy, the body's built-in cellular cleanup process.

This is why fasting has always been more than a religious practice. It is a Kingdom pattern for restoration. Spirit, soul, and body all benefit when you make room for God and bring your appetites back under His leadership.

**FASTING IS ONE OF GOD'S GIFTS FOR RENEWAL,
HELPING YOU QUIET THE FLESH, SHARPEN DISCERNMENT,
AND MAKE ROOM FOR HEALING.**

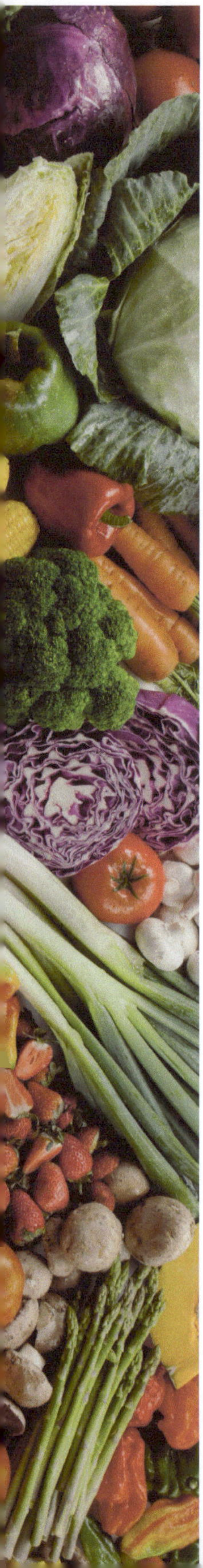

7X TIPS

TIP 1: GOOD MORNING, HOLY SPIRIT!

Before you get out of bed, pause and say, "Good morning, Holy Spirit. What would you have me do today?"

Then listen. Before your feet hit the floor, take a moment to pray, meditate on your scripture of the day, and take a few deep breaths. Let your first thoughts belong to God.

TIP 2: WATER LOAD

Begin your day with 12 to 20 ounces of purified water, with lemon if desired. Your daily goal is to drink half your body weight in ounces throughout the day. Give your body the hydration it needs before reaching for anything else.

TIP 3: OPTIMIZE YOUR FUEL

Follow the weekly 7X food plan as closely as possible. Choose clean, whole foods that nourish your body and support healing. Focus on vegetables, quality proteins, healthy fats, and fruit in moderation. When possible, choose foods that are organic, pasture-raised, and close to their natural state.

TIP 4: PRAY

When hunger rises, do not panic. Pause and pray. Use that moment to seek God, quiet your flesh, and invite the Holy Spirit into your cravings. Hunger can become a reminder to turn your attention back to Him.

TIP 5: HUMILITY & GRATITUDE

Do not make this challenge about appearances or attention. Let this be a private act of worship between you and the Father. Stay humble. Stay thankful. At the end of each day, thank God for at least one way He strengthened or provided for you.

"But when you fast, put oil on your head and wash your face, so that it will not be obvious to others that you are fasting, but only to your Father, who is unseen; and your Father, who sees what is done in secret, will reward you."
— Matthew 6:17-18

Before you go to sleep, take one quiet moment to thank God for your blessings and give thanks for at least one thing that happened during your day.

DANIEL FAST EXPLAINED

One of the clearest biblical examples of intentional eating and spiritual conviction is found in the book of Daniel.

Daniel was a young Hebrew taken captive into Babylon and selected for training in the king's palace. As part of that training, he and the other young men were offered the finest food and wine in the empire. But Daniel recognized that this was about more than food. It was about consecration, discernment, and obedience.

Scripture says:

"Daniel resolved not to defile himself with the royal food and wine."
— Daniel 1:8

So Daniel made a request. Instead of eating the rich food from the king's table, he asked for vegetables and water. This was a bold act of conviction, especially because the official responsible for him could have faced serious consequences if Daniel appeared weak or unhealthy.

Daniel proposed a test:

"Please test your servants for ten days: Give us nothing but vegetables to eat and water to drink. Then compare our appearance with that of the young men who eat the royal food."
— Daniel 1:12–13

Ten days later, the results were unmistakable:

"At the end of the ten days they looked healthier and better nourished than any of the young men who ate the royal food."
— Daniel 1:15

Daniel and his friends were not only physically stronger. They were mentally sharper and spiritually grounded.

The story of Daniel is not merely about vegetables. It is about choosing what is pure over what is indulgent, what is life-giving over what is excessive, and what honors God over what simply satisfies the flesh.

Thousands of years later, the same choice still stands before us.

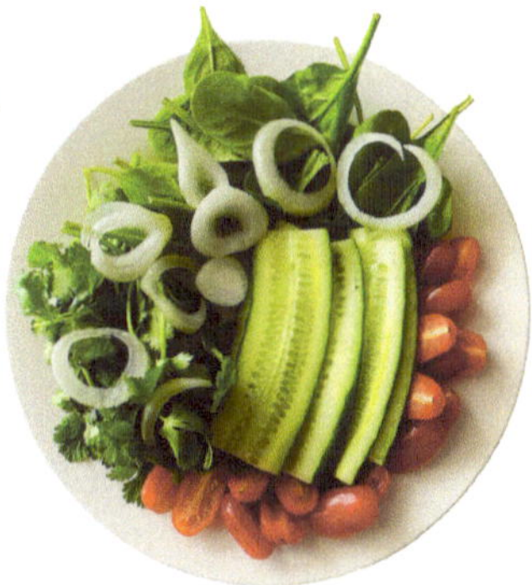

Every day, we are presented with two tables.
One offers convenience, engineering, and indulgence.
The other offers what is clean, nourishing, and life-giving.

The question is the same one Daniel faced:

Which table will you choose?

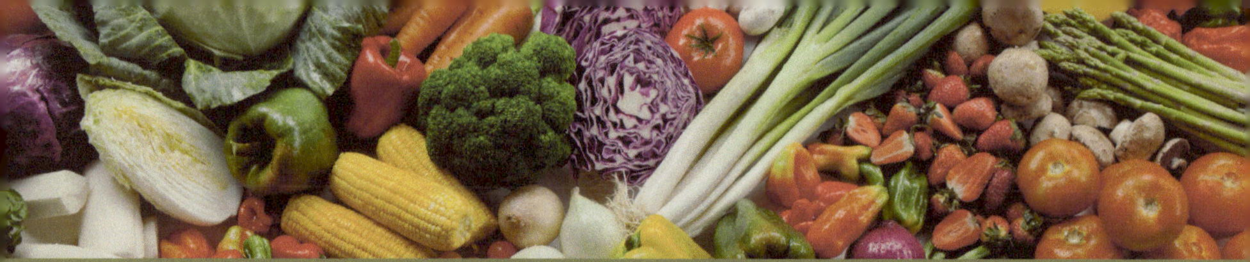

DANIEL FAST
WITH OPTIONAL DETOX

BEFORE YOU BEGIN

- This fast may trigger temporary detox symptoms such as headaches, fatigue, light-headedness, or flu-like discomfort. Do not be alarmed. As your body begins releasing stored toxins, rest well, drink plenty of water, and move through the process with patience.

- If you are using the juicing recipes, note that they are written for two people. If you are juicing for one, simply cut the recipes in half.

- Eliminate alcohol, sugar, processed foods, and white flour products during this phase.

- Optional juices may be included as part of this fast.

- Drink half your body weight in ounces of water each day. Filtered or purified water is best. You may add fresh lemon to increase your body's alkalinity, if desired.

- Herbal teas are permitted.

- Practice deep breathing techniques. First, take a normal breath. Then take a deep breath: Breathe in slowly through your nose, allowing your chest and lower belly to rise as you fill your lungs. Concentrate on taking in the presence of God. Pause for three seconds. Let your abdomen expand fully. Now breathe out slowly through your mouth and focus on releasing all anxiety, unforgiveness, negative energy, and toxins.

- Choose the cleanest food sources available to you. When possible, select organic, in-season, and locally grown produce.

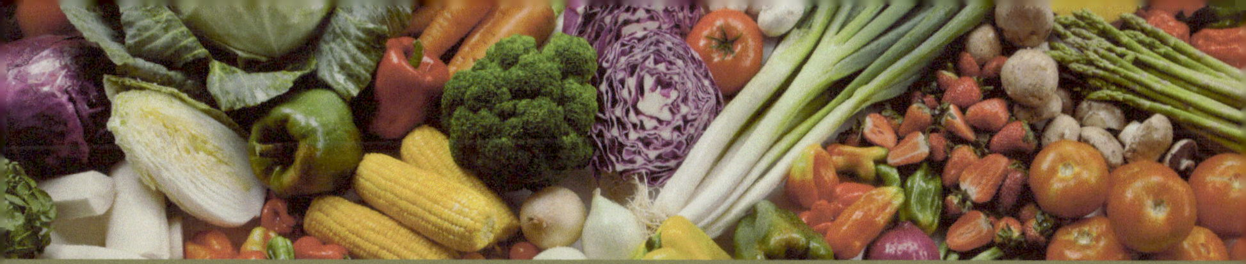

DANIEL FAST
WITH OPTIONAL DETOX

This suggested grocery list supports the recipes and detox options in the Daniel Fast section. Use it as a guide and adjust based on your preferences, household needs, and availability in your area.

- Filtered, reverse osmosis water or alkaline water
- Raw, organic, and unsalted walnuts, pecans, and almonds
- Apples or green apples
- Pears
- Nectarines
- Cantaloupe
- Ripe bananas
- Lemons
- Carrots
- Cucumbers
- Celery
- Spinach
- Kale
- Swiss chard
- Bok choy
- Parsley
- Fresh cilantro
- Red beets with stems
- Broccoli
- Cabbage
- Zucchini

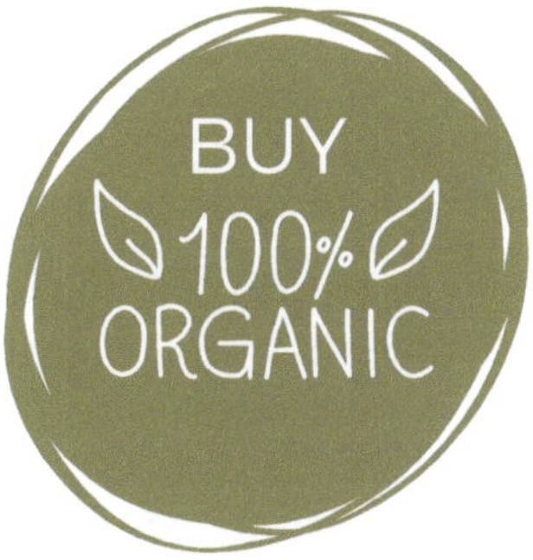

- Tomatoes
- Onions
- Garlic
- Ginger
- Daikon radish
- Brown rice
- Dried white beans
- Chia seeds
- Almond meal
- Bay leaves
- Cayenne pepper
- Ground cinnamon
- Sea salt
- Turmeric
- Extra virgin olive oil
- Organic coconut oil
- • Miso
- Baking soda
- Vegetable stock
- Organic castor oil
- Honey

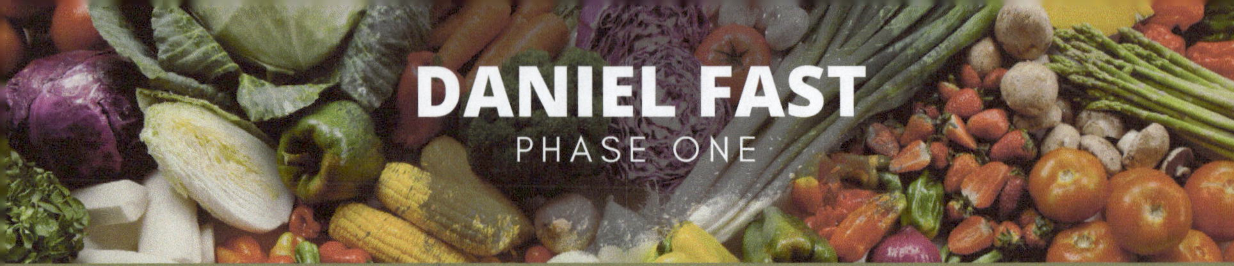

DANIEL FAST

PHASE ONE

DAYS 1-3 (CLEANSE)

STEP 1: GOOD MORNING, HOLY SPIRIT!

Before you get out of bed, say, "Good morning, Holy Spirit. What would You have me do today?" Pause, listen, and take a few deep breaths. Before your feet hit the floor, meditate on your scripture of the day and surrender your thoughts to God.

STEP 2: WATER LOAD

Begin your day with 12 to 20 ounces of purified water, with lemon if desired. Work toward your daily goal of drinking half your body weight in ounces of water.

STEP 3: MORNING GLORY

5 carrots
1/2 green apple
4 ounces of spinach and parsley
4 stalks of celery
1/2 red beet with stem
1 cucumber

Suggested substitutions: Kale, Swiss chard, cabbage, bok choy, or endive may be used in place of the greens listed above.

Optional add-ins: 1/2 lemon, a small piece of ginger root, or 5 walnuts may be added to selected recipes if desired.

Preparation: Thoroughly wash ingredients and run through a juicer.

Optional note: If needed, you may also have 1/2 cup raw organic unsalted pecans or almonds, or one piece of raw organic fruit such as an apple, pear, nectarine, or cantaloupe.

STEP 4: MID-DAY BOOST

5 Carrots
1 Small Apple (of choice)
1" slice of Ginger
½ root Turmeric
1 ½ cups Spinach
½ Lemon

STEP 5: EVENING TONIC

5 carrots
1/2 green apple
3 stalks of celery
4 ounces of broccoli and spinach
1 beet with stem
1 cucumber
1-inch piece of ginger root

STEP 6: PRAYER

Throughout the day, when hunger rises, pause and pray. Ask God for wisdom, strength, and deeper discipline. Let every craving become an invitation to seek Him first.

STEP 7: HUMILITY & GRATITUDE

Before bed, take a moment to thank God for at least one way He met you today. Stay humble, stay thankful, and let this fast remain a private act of worship before the Lord.

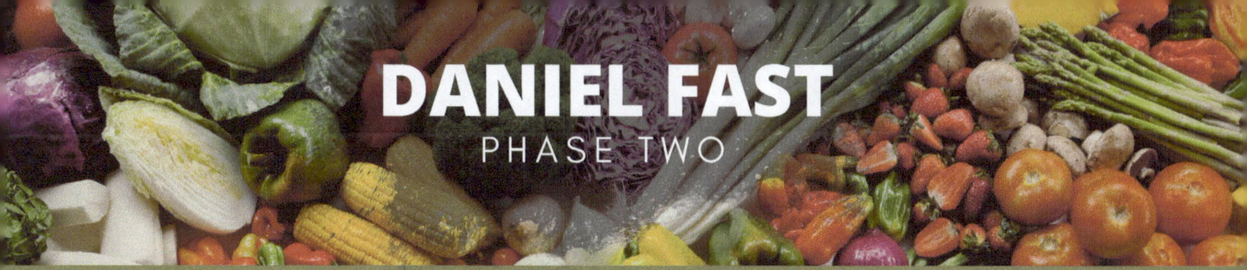

DANIEL FAST
PHASE TWO

DAYS 4 -18

You made it through the first three days. That matters. By now, your body is beginning to adjust, your cravings may be calming, and your discipline is getting stronger.

During this phase, you will continue the foundational rhythms from Phase One while adding salads, vegetable soups, and simple whole-food meals. Keep it clean, prayerful, and consistent.

DAILY FLOW

1. **GOOD MORNING, HOLY SPIRIT!**
   Begin your day with prayer, surrender, and a posture of listening.

2. **WATER LOAD**
   Continue drinking half your body weight in ounces of water each day.

3. **MORNING GLORY JUICE**
   Start your day with one of the juices from Phase One.

4. **MID-MORNING SNACK**
   Choose from raw nuts, fruit, raw vegetables, or one of the approved options on the recipe page.

5. **LUNCH**
   Eat a large salad with a variety of dark leafy greens and raw vegetables. Use organic balsamic vinaigrette or another clean dressing. (No cheese or croutons.)

6. **AFTERNOON SNACK**
   Choose from raw nuts, fruit, raw vegetables, or one of the approved recipe options.

7. **DINNER**
   Eat another large salad or choose one of the suggested soup recipes.

8. **PRAYER**
   Throughout the day, when hunger rises or your flesh gets loud, pause and pray. Give God your attention, and let every craving become a cue to seek Him first.

9. **HUMILITY AND GRATITUDE**
   Before bed, take a moment to thank God for how He carried you through the day. Stay humble, stay prayerful, and let this fast remain a private act of worship.

"If my people, who are called by my name, will humble themselves and pray and seek my face... then I will hear from heaven... "
— 2 Chronicles 7:14

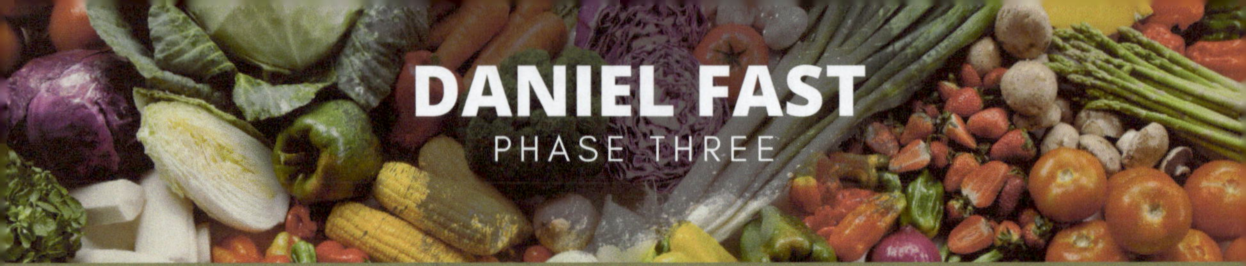

DANIEL FAST

PHASE THREE

DAYS 19-21

WATER FAST

The final three days of your Daniel Fast are a sacred invitation to go deeper. This phase is designed to quiet the flesh, sharpen your focus, and help you give greater attention to the voice of the Holy Spirit.

A 3-day water fast can also provide the body with a meaningful metabolic reset. As your digestive system rests, your body can redirect energy toward repair, cleansing, and renewal.

This is about consecration.
This is about surrender.
This is about making room for God.

If you are taking blood sugar medication, have a medical condition, or have any concerns about fasting, consult your physician before beginning a complete water fast.

During these three days:

- Continue prayer and scripture meditation.
- Drink plenty of water.
- Rest as needed.
- Keep your schedule lighter if possible.
- Pay attention to what God is revealing.

What to expect:

You may notice moments of hunger, fatigue, irritability, or mental resistance, especially in the beginning. Stay calm. Slow down. Drink water. Pray through the discomfort. Let weakness become an invitation to depend more deeply on God.

You may also experience greater clarity, lighter digestion, increased spiritual sensitivity, and a deeper awareness of the Holy Spirit's leading. Do not rush these days. Let them be quiet, reverent, and intentional.

"Man shall not live by bread alone, but by every word that proceeds from the mouth of God."
— Matthew 4:4

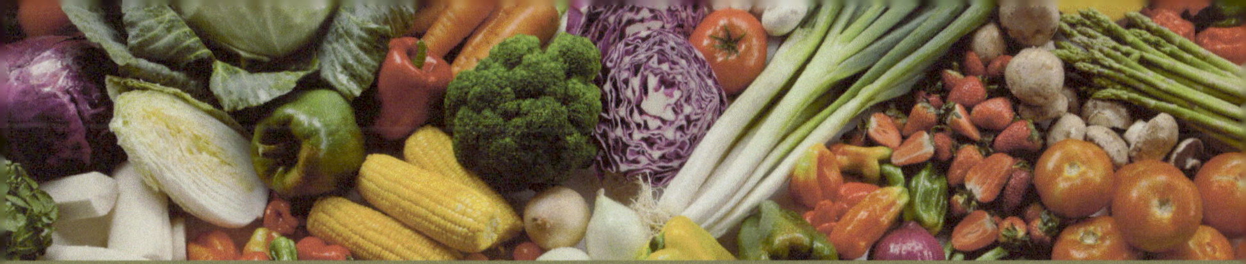

MORE CLEANSING SUPPORT
CLEANSE TO HEAL

These optional practices may support your body's natural detox pathways during the Daniel Fast. Use wisdom, listen to your body, and choose only what feels appropriate for your health and season.

DRY BRUSHING

Known to help stimulate circulation, support lymphatic flow, and encourage the body's natural cleansing process.

1. Using a natural-bristle brush or loofah, gently brush the skin in upward strokes, moving from the feet toward the heart.
2. Brush the arms toward the chest and collarbone area, where major lymph drainage occurs.
3. Dry brush for 5 to 10 minutes, 1 to 2 times per day.

LYMPHATIC PUMP

Gentle movement and muscle contraction can help support the lymphatic system, which plays a key role in moving waste out of the body.

1. Tighten and release the muscles of the legs, core, and arms in sequence, holding each contraction for about 5 seconds and releasing for 5 seconds.
2. Repeat several times for each muscle group.
3. A mini-trampoline or gentle rebounding for 5 to 15 minutes may also help stimulate lymphatic flow.

CASTOR OIL BATH

1. Castor oil has traditionally been used to support relaxation and the body's natural cleansing process through the skin.
2. Three times per week, massage the skin from head to toe with a mixture of equal parts organic olive oil and cold-pressed castor oil.
3. Allow the oil to remain on the skin while soaking in a warm bath for 15 minutes. After the bath, wrap up warmly, rest for up to an hour if desired, and then shower.

OPTIONAL DIGESTIVE SUPPORT
Some people choose to use Mag07 or a similar cleanser.

Take 2 tablets in the morning on an empty stomach with 12 ounces of water.

Supports:

- healthy digestion
- regular elimination
- relief from occasional constipation

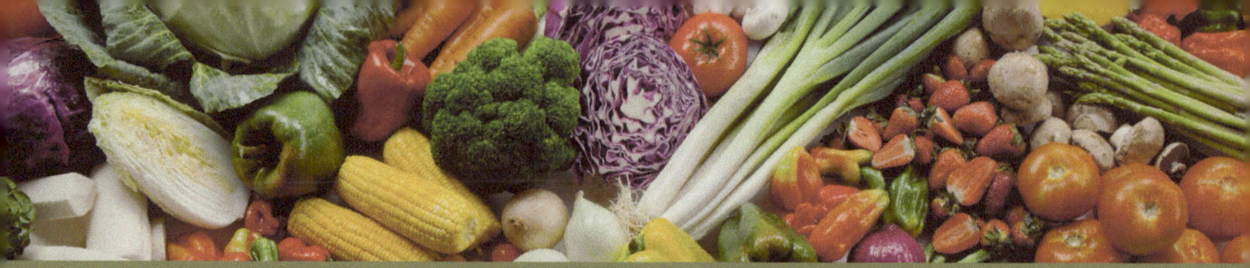

CHALLENGE SUPPORT FOODS

These recipes are included to support you during the 7X Challenge. They are not meant to become comfort foods or substitutes for surrender. Use them with wisdom and only when needed for nourishment, steadiness, and strength. The goal is not indulgence. The goal is alignment.

ORGANIC ITALIAN VEGETABLE SOUP

Ingredients:

- 1 cup dried white beans, or a combination of dried beans
- 3 quarts vegetable stock or water
- 1/4 cup extra virgin olive oil
- 2 onions, sliced
- 2 stalks of celery, sliced
- 2 large zucchini, sliced (optional)
- 2 to 3 medium fresh tomatoes, chopped
- 1 to 2 cloves garlic, minced
- 1 small head of cabbage, thinly sliced
- 4 to 5 medium carrots, sliced
- 1 cup daikon radish, cubed
- 1/2 cup fresh parsley
- 1/2 cup brown rice
- 3 bay leaves
- 1 package miso
- Cayenne pepper to taste

Instructions

Place the beans in a large bowl and cover with water by at least one inch. Soak overnight, then drain. Add the soaked beans to a large soup pot with the stock or water. Bring to a boil, then reduce the heat, cover, and simmer for about 1 hour.

In a separate skillet, heat the olive oil and sauté the onions until softened. Add the celery, zucchini, garlic, and fresh tomatoes. Simmer for 20 minutes. Add the cabbage, carrots, radish, parsley, brown rice, bay leaves, miso, cayenne, and sautéed vegetables to the soup pot. Cover and simmer until the rice is tender and the vegetables are cooked through.

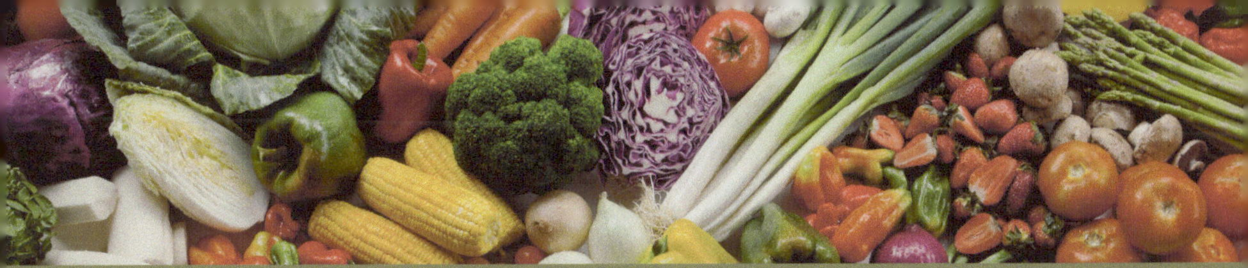

THE EPIPHANY SMOOTHIE

Ingredients:

- 1 cup nut milk or water
- 1 ripe pear
- 2 handfuls of fresh spinach
- 1/2 avocado
- 1/2 avocado seed
- Small piece of fresh ginger, grated
- 1/2 apple

Instructions

Blend all ingredients until smooth.

Note: Avocado is rich in healthy fats, fiber, and antioxidants, making this smoothie a nourishing support option during the challenge.

PALEO BANANA NUT MUFFINS (FOR ADDED SUSTENANCE)

Ingredients:

- 3 cups almond meal
- 2 t baking soda
- 1/2 t salt
- 4 T coconut oil
- 2 T chia seeds,
- 2 ripe bananas, mashed
- 1 T vanilla extract
- 1 T ground cinnamon
- 4 T honey

Instructions

Preheat the oven to 350°F.

Mix chia seeds with water and place in the fridge for 15 minutes.

Combine all ingredients, except for the chia seed mix, in a large bowl. Once combined, add the chia seed mix and combine everything to form a batter. Spoon the batter into the muffin tin and smooth the tops with the spoon. Bake for 15 minutes, or until lightly golden brown on top. Place a skewer in the center of a muffin, and if it comes out clean, it's ready. Remove from the oven and allow muffins to cool in the tray.

Support foods are not shortcuts. They are tools to help you stay the course with wisdom.

YOU DID IT!

Congratulations! You have completed the **Fueled 7X Challenge.**

For the past 49 days, you have practiced intentional choices that strengthen the body, renew the mind, and align the spirit. You have not just followed a plan. You have begun building a new pattern of life.

That is what real transformation looks like.

Lasting change is rarely created in a single dramatic moment. It is formed through repeated decisions. One prayer at a time. One fast at a time. One meal at a time. One surrendered choice at a time.

This challenge was never just about weight loss or willpower. It was about becoming the kind of person who lives with greater clarity, discipline, obedience, and peace.

Now the question is not, "Did it work?"
The question is, "Who are you becoming?"

You are becoming someone who pauses before reacting.
Someone who listens before consuming.
Someone who chooses life over impulse.
Someone who honors God in body, mind, and spirit.

Do not underestimate what these 49 days have built in you.

The habits you repeat will shape the life you live. So keep going. You did not come this far to return to what once ruled you. Protect what God has built in you, and keep walking in the life that leads to peace.

Small choices, repeated with consistency, become a strong life.

Goal: To reflect God daily in every area of your life.

"Do not grow weary in doing good, for at the proper time
you will reap a harvest if you do not give up."
— Galatians 6:9

FAQS

Q1: What exactly is the Fueled 7X Challenge?

A: The Fueled 7X Challenge is a 7-week, 49-day journey of spiritual focus, physical renewal, and intentional lifestyle change. It is not just a diet or fitness plan. It is a practical way to apply the 7 Pillars of Optimal Wellness and align your body, mind, and spirit with God's design.

Q2: What should I do before I begin?

A: Begin prayerfully. Review the challenge materials, prepare your food and supplies, and set your heart with intention. You may also want to take a "before" photo, write down your goals, and make space in your schedule for rest, reflection, and consistency.

Q3: What is the Daniel Fast during this challenge?

A: The Daniel Fast takes place during Weeks 4 through 6 and focuses on simple, whole foods such as fruits, vegetables, seeds, nuts, and water. It is a time of consecration, cleansing, prayer, and deeper dependence on God.

Q4: What is the 3-Day Water Fast at the end of Week 6?

A: At the end of Week 6, the challenge moves into a 3-day water fast for those who can participate. This phase is designed to deepen surrender, sharpen spiritual focus, and give the body a time of rest and reset.

Q5: Can I modify the fast if I have medical concerns?

A: Yes. If you have a diagnosed medical condition, are pregnant, nursing, taking medication, or have other health concerns, consult your doctor before beginning any fast. If needed, choose a modified version that supports your health needs. The goal is wisdom, not pressure.

Q6: What if I get hungry during the challenge?

A: Hunger is part of the process, especially in the early days. Before reacting, pause. Drink water. Pray. Ask whether your body needs nourishment or whether your flesh is resisting change. Use support foods with wisdom when needed, but do not let discomfort pull you back into old patterns.

Q7: What if I mess up during the challenge?

A: Do not quit. Do not move into shame. Acknowledge it, reset, and keep going. This challenge is not about perfection. It is about humility, consistency, and learning how to realign quickly when you get off course.

Q8: Do I need to complete every part perfectly for it to count?

A: No. The goal is not flawless performance. The goal is willing obedience, intentional alignment, and steady progress. God honors a surrendered heart.

Remember: this challenge is not about earning God's love. It is about aligning your life with His wisdom.

FUELED

FOR THE HOLIDAYS

10 TIPS FOR STAYING ON TRACK DURING THE HOLIDAYS

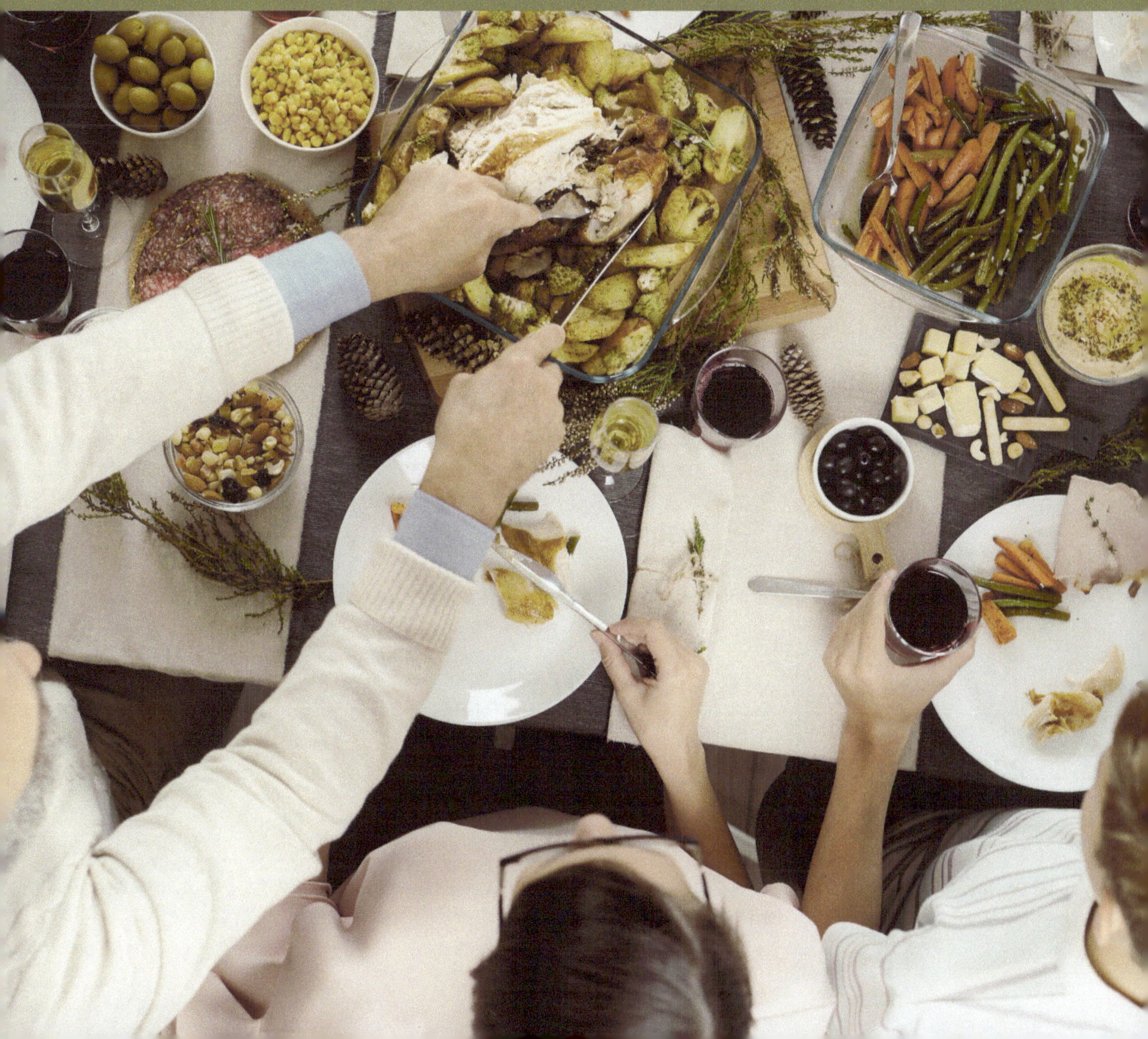

10 TIPS FOR STAYING ON TRACK DURING THE HOLIDAYS

The holiday season brings joy, celebration, and, let's be honest, more sweets, stress, and schedule overload than almost any other time of year. But a full calendar and a loaded dessert table do not have to pull you off course. The 7 Pillars of Optimal Wellness can help you stay grounded, energized, and aligned with God through every gathering, meal, and moment. Here are 10 Faith-Fueled ways to move through the holidays with confidence, clarity, and peace.

1. START WITH YOUR SPIRIT

"Seek first the kingdom of God and His righteousness,
and all these things shall be added to you."
— Matthew 6:33

Before the day gets busy, begin with God. Invite the Holy Spirit into your day, schedule, conversations, and cravings. A Spirit-led morning leads to Spirit-led choices.

2. GUARD YOUR MIND

"Let every person be quick to hear, slow to speak, slow to anger."
— James 1:19

Crowded schedules and tense conversations can test your patience. Decide in advance that you are not there to win arguments. You are there to walk in grace.

3. HYDRATE ON PURPOSE

"Whoever drinks the water I give them will never thirst."
— John 4:14

Water may not feel festive, but it is one of the simplest ways to stay clear, energized, and in control. Staying hydrated helps curb cravings, supports energy, and gives your body what it actually needs. Carry your water and lemon like it is part of your life, because it is.

4. PLAN TO WINç

"So whether you eat or drink, or whatever you do, do all to the glory of God."
— 1 Corinthians 10:31

Do not show up overly hungry. Eat something balanced before gatherings so you are not making decisions from depletion. Focus on protein, fiber, and whole foods first.

5. PROTECT YOUR REST

"He gives His beloved sleep."
— Psalm 127:2

Late nights may feel festive, but rest is still holy. When you are well-rested, you think more clearly, respond with more patience, and stay stronger in every area.

6. KEEP MOVING, EVEN JUST A LITTLE

"Physical training is of some value..."
— 1 Timothy 4:8

You do not need a perfect workout to stay aligned. Take a brisk walk, stretch between tasks, or move while dinner is cooking. Small movement still matters.

7. PAUSE WITH PURPOSE

"Be still, and know that I am God."
— Psalm 46:10

Before you go back for seconds, say yes to one more event, or react emotionally, pause. A few quiet seconds with the Holy Spirit can realign your heart and choices.

8. SET BOUNDARIES WITH BOLDNESS AND GRACE

"Let your 'Yes' be yes and your 'No' be no."
— Matthew 5:37

You do not have to say yes to every invitation, every expectation, or every plate put in front of you. Boundaries protect your peace, health, and focus.

9. SOAK IN GRATITUDE

"Give thanks in all circumstances..."
— 1 Thessalonians 5:18

The holidays are about presence, not perfection. Gratitude shifts your focus from what is missing to what God is already doing.

10. WEEKLY RESET RITUALS

"Examine yourselves... "
— 2 Corinthians 13:5

Take a few minutes each week to reflect. Where did you stay aligned? Where did you drift? Celebrate the wins, make the adjustments, and keep going.

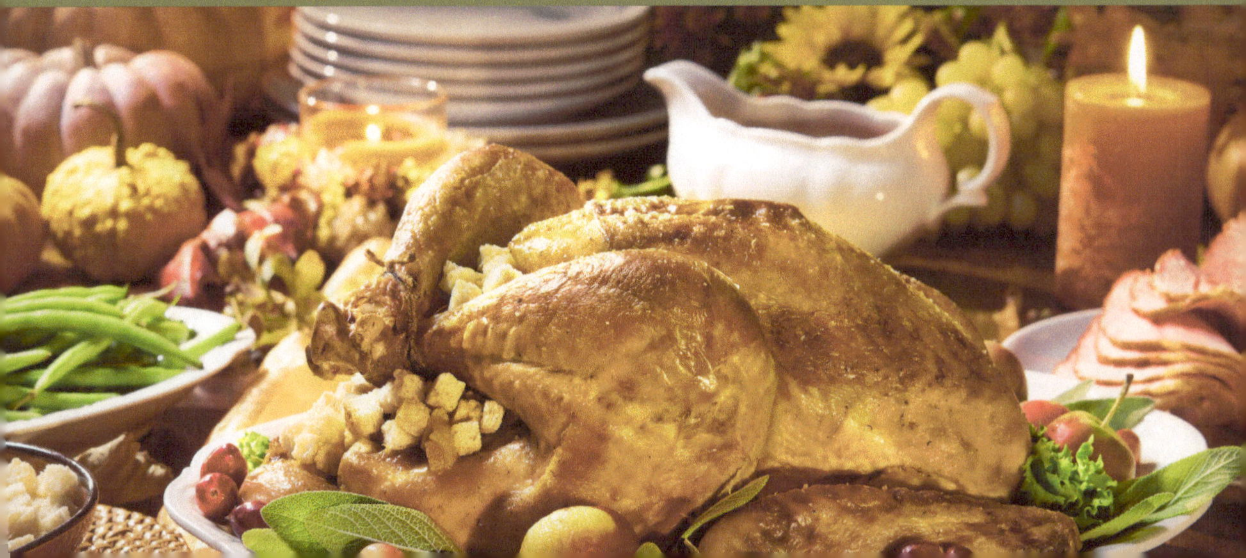

NOTES:

Chapter 3: Hydration

1.Ostrowska, J., & Szostak-Węgierek, D. (2025). *The Influence of Body Composition and Lifestyle Factors on Resting Energy Expenditure and Its Role in Cardiometabolic Risk: A Cross-Sectional Study.*https://doi.org/10.20944/preprints202501.1442.v1

2.Shekarforoush, S., & Fardaee, M. (2020). *The effects of hydration status on cardiovascular system: a review.* 3(2), 9–14. http://fh.srbiau.ac.ir/article_16024.html

3.Vlastos, G. A., Tangney, C. C., & Rosenson, R. S. (2003). *Effects of hydration on blood rheology.* Clinical Hemorheology and Microcirculation, 28(1), 41–49. https://content.iospress.com/articles/clinical-hemorheology-and-microcirculation/ch535

4.Lieberman, H. R. (2010). *Hydration and Human Cognition.* Nutrition Today, 45*(6).* https://doi.org/10.1097/NT.0B013E3181FE1747

5.D'Anci, K. E. (2011). *Hydration and mental performance. (pp. 180–193).* Woodhead Publishing Ltd. https://doi.org/10.1533/9780857092922.2.180

6.Wongta, A. (2025). *Respiratory health and chronic disease risks in residents of agricultural areas in Chiang Mai, Northern Thailand.* https://doi.org/10.1371/journal.pone.0321471

7.Filardo, S., Scalese, G., Virili, C., Pontone, S., Di Pietro, M., Covelli, A. S., Bedetti, G., Marinelli, P., Bruno, G., Stramazzo, I., Centanni, M., Sessa, R., & Severi, C. (2022). *The Potential Role of Hypochlorhydria in the Development of Duodenal Dysbiosis: A Preliminary Report.* Frontiers in Cellular and Infection Microbiology, 12. https://doi.org/10.3389/fcimb.2022.854904

8.Sarker, S. A., Ahmed, T., & Brüssow, H. (2017). *Hunger and microbiology: is a low gastric acid-induced bacterial overgrowth in the small intestine a contributor to malnutrition in developing countries?* Microbial Biotechnology, *10*(5), 1025–1030.https://doi.org/10.1111/1751-7915.12780

9.Ignacio, R. M. C., Joo, K.-B., & Lee, K.-J. (2020). *Clinical Effect and Mechanism of Alkaline Reduced Water.* Journal of Food and Drug Analysis, *20*(1), 394–397. https://doi.org/10.38212/2224-6614.2099

10.Hu, D., Kabayama, S., Watanabe, Y., & Cui, Y. (2024). Health Benefits of Electrolyzed Hydrogen Water: Antioxidant and Anti-Inflammatory Effects in Living Organisms. Antioxidants. https://doi.org/10.3390/antiox13030313

11.Meng, F., Liu, Z., Qin, S., & Liu, B. (2025). Oral Administration of Hydrogen-rich Water: Biomedical Activities, Potential Mechanisms, and Clinical Applications. Current Pharmaceutical Design, 31. https://doi.org/10.2174/0113816128330516241121150719

12.Yaghoubi, A., Soleimanpour, S., & Avan, A. (2024). Hydrogen-Rich Water Using as a Modulator of Gut Microbiota and Managing the Inflammatory Bowel Disease (pp. 261–286). Springer International Publishing. https://doi.org/10.1007/978-3-031-47375-3_17

13.Abol-Enein, H., Gheith, O., Barakat, N., Nour, E. M., & Sharaf, A.-E. (2009). Ionized Alkaline Water: New Strategy for Management of Metabolic Acidosis in Experimental Animals. Therapeutic Apheresis and Dialysis, 13(3), 220–224. https://doi.org/10.1111/J.1744-9987.2009.00659.X

14.Nimone, S. B., Goukonde, R., & Sanap, G. (2025). RO Water Effect on Human Body. International Journal of Advanced Research in Science, Communication and Technology, 538–548. https://doi.org/10.48175/ijarsct-22956

15.Rosborg, I., Kozisek, F., & Ferrrante, M. (2015). Health effects of demineralization drinking water (pp. 119–123). Springer. https://doi.org/10.1007/978-3-319-09593-6_7

NOTES:

Chapter 4: Nutrition

1.Naude, D. F. (2022). *Chronic Sub-Clinical Systemic Metabolic Acidosis – A Review with Implications for Clinical Practice.* Journal of Evidence-Based Integrative Medicine, 27. https://doi.org/10.1177/2515690X221142352

2.Álvarez-Herms, J. (2024). *Summatory Effects of Anaerobic Exercise and a 'Westernized Athletic Diet' on Gut Dysbiosis and Chronic Low-Grade Metabolic Acidosis*. Microorganisms, 12(6), 1138. https://doi.org/10.3390/microorganisms12061138

3.Wieërs, M., Beynon-Cobb, B., Visser, W. J., & Attaye, I. (2024). *Dietary acid load in health and disease. Pflügers Archiv: European Journal of Physiology.* https://doi.org/10.1007/s00424-024-02910-7

4.Amodu, A., & Abramowitz, M. K. (2016). *Effects of Metabolic Acidosis on Skeletal Muscle* In Acid-base disorders and their treatment (pp. 101–110)pp. 101–110). Springer, New York, NY. https://doi.org/10.1007/978-1-4939-3463-8_10

5.Siri-Tarino, P. W., Sun, Q., Hu, F. B., & Krauss, R. M. (2010). *Meta-analysis of prospective cohort studies evaluating the association of saturated fat with cardiovascular disease*. The American journal of clinical nutrition, 91(3), 535–546.

6.Crick, D. C., Halligan, S., Davey Smith, G., Khandaker, G., & Jones, H. J. (2023). *Relationship between Polyunsaturated Fatty Acids and Inflammation: evidence from cohort and Mendelian randomization analyses*. medRxiv.

7.DiNicolantonio, J. J., & O'Keefe, J. H. (2018). *Importance of maintaining a low omega–6/omega–3 ratio for reducing inflammation. 5*(2). https://doi.org/10.1136/OPENHRT-2018-000946

8.Simopoulos, A. P. (2016). *An Increase in the Omega-6/Omega-3 Fatty Acid Ratio Increases the Risk for Obesity*. Nutrients, 8(3), 128. https://doi.org/10.3390/NU8030128

9.Noori, N., Dukkipati, R., Kovesdy, C. P., Kovesdy, C. P., Sim, J. J., Feroze, U., Murali, S. B., Bross, R., Benner, D., Kopple, J. D., Kalantar-Zadeh, K., & Kalantar-Zadeh, K. (2011). Dietary Omega-3 Fatty Acid, Ratio of Omega-6 to Omega-3 Intake, Inflammation, and Survival in Long-term Hemodialysis Patients. American Journal of Kidney Diseases, 58(2), 248–256. https://doi.org/10.1053/J.AJKD.2011.03.017

10.Dietary Fat Myths & Cardiovascular Risk
Kendrick, M. (2007). The great cholesterol con: The truth about what really causes heart disease and how to avoid it. John Blake Publishing.

11.Hooper, L., Abdelhamid, A., Bunn, D., Brown, T., & Summerbell, C. D. (2015). Reduced or modified dietary fat for preventing cardiovascular disease. Cochrane Database of Systematic Reviews, 2015(6), CD011737.

12.Astrup, A., Teicholz, N., Magkos, F., Bier, D. M., Brenna, J. T., King, J. C., Mente, A., Ordovas, J. M., Volek, J. S., Yusuf, S., & Krauss, R. M. (2021). Dietary Saturated Fats and Health: Are the U.S. Guidelines Evidence-Based?. Nutrients, 13(10), 3305.

13.Heileson, J. L. (2020). *Dietary saturated fat and heart disease: A narrative review*. Nutrition Reviews, *78*(6), 474–485._

NOTES:

14.Johannesen, C. D. L., Langsted, A., Mortensen, M. B., & Nordestgaard, B. G. (2020). *Association between low density lipoprotein and all-cause and cause-specific mortality in Denmark: Prospective cohort study.* BMJ, 371, Article *m4266*.
https://doi.org/10.1136/bmj.m4266
15.Hyman, M. (2021). *The Pegan diet: 21 practical principles for reclaiming your health in a nutritionally confusing world*. Little, Brown Spark.
16.Hwang, H.-J., Liu, Y., Kim, H.-S., Lee, H., Lim, Y., & Park, H. (2019). *Daily walnut intake improves metabolic syndrome status and increases circulating adiponectin levels: randomized controlled crossover trial.* Nutrition Research and Practice, 13(2), 105–114.
https://doi.org/10.4162/NRP.2019.13.2.105
17.Dutta, S., & Mitra, R. (2025). *Effects of walnut consumption on brain health: A review.* Journal of Current Research in Food Science, 6(1a), Article 180.
https://doi.org/10.22271/foodsci.2025.v6.i1a.180
18.Rajaram, S., Valls-Pedret, C., Cofán, M., et al. (2017). The Walnuts and Healthy Aging Study (WAHA): Protocol for a nutritional intervention trial with walnuts on brain aging. Frontiers in Aging Neuroscience, 8, Article 333.
19.Samra, M., & Gupta, I. (2024). From smoothies to dialysis: The impact of oxalate nephropathy. Cureus, 16(8), e67409.
https://doi.org/10.7759/cureus.67409
20.Taylor, E. N., & Curhan, G. C. (2007). Oxalate intake and the risk for nephropathy. Journal of the American Society of Nephrology, 18(7), 2198–2204. https://doi.org/10.1681/ASN.2007020219
21.Novitasari, E., & Savage, G. P. (2021). Oxalate contents in green juice prepared using either a high-speed blender or a masticating juicer. E3S Web of Conferences, 306, 04004.
https://doi.org/10.1051/E3SCONF/202130604004
22.Chew, B. H., Lange, D., & Sutton, R. A. L. (2012). Oxalate and urolithiasis. In M. Khan (Ed.), Kidney Stone Disease (pp. 315–329). Springer.https://doi.org/10.1007/978-1-4471-4387-1_19
23.Grentz, L. M., & Massey, L. K. (2002). Contribution of dietary oxalate to urinary oxalate in health and disease. Topics in Clinical Nutrition, 17(2), 64–70. https://doi.org/10.1097/00008486-200203000-00010
24.Kuhnt, K., Wagner, A., Kraft, J., Basu, S., & Jahreis, G. (2006). Dietary supplementation with 11trans- and 12trans-18:1 and oxidative stress in humans. The American Journal of Clinical Nutrition, 84(5), 981–988. https://doi.org/10.1093/AJCN/84.5.981
25.Hirata, Y. (2021). Trans-Fatty acids as an enhancer of inflammation and cell death: Molecular basis for their pathological actions. Biological & Pharmaceutical Bulletin, 44(10), 1487–1495.
26.Serreli, G., Boronat, A., de la Torre, R., Rodríguez-Morató, J., & Deiana, M. (2024). *Cardiovascular and metabolic benefits of extra virgin olive oil phenolic compounds: Mechanistic insights from in vivo studies*. Cells, 13(18), 1555. https://doi.org/10.3390/cells13181555
27.Millman, J. F., Okamoto, S., Teruya, T., Uema, T., Ikematsu, S., Shimabukuro, M., & Masuzaki, H. (2021). *Extra-virgin olive oil and the gut-brain axis: Influence on gut microbiota, mucosal immunity, and cardiometabolic and cognitive health.* Nutrition Reviews, 79(6), 814–828.
https://doi.org/10.1093/nutrit/nuaa148
28.Flynn, M. M., Tierney, A. C., & Itsiopoulos, C. (2023). Is extra virgin olive oil the critical ingredient driving the health benefits of a Mediterranean diet? A narrative review. Nutrients, 15(13), 2916.
https://doi.org/10.3390/nu15132916

NOTES:

29.Virruso, C., Accardi, G., Colonna-Romano, G., Candore, G., Vasto, S., & Caruso, C. (2014). *Nutraceutical properties of extra-virgin olive oil: A natural remedy for age-related disease?* Rejuvenation Research, 17(2), 217–224. https://doi.org/10.1089/rej.2013.1532

30.Lombardo, L., Grasso, F., Lanciano, F., Loria, S., & Monetti, E. (2018). *Broad-spectrum health protection of extra virgin olive oil compounds.* In Olive Oil – Constituents, Quality, Health Properties and Bioconversions (pp. 27–48). Elsevier.

31.van Vliet, S., Bain, J. R., Muehlbauer, M. J., Provenza, F. D., Kronberg, S. L., Pieper, C. F., & Huffman, K. M. (2021). *A metabolomics comparison of plant-based meat and grass-fed meat indicates large nutritional differences despite comparable Nutrition Facts panels.* Scientific Reports, 11, 13828. https://doi.org/10.1038/s41598-021-93100-3

32.Krusinski, L., Sergin, S., Jambunathan, V., Rowntree, J. E., & Fenton, J. I. (2022). *Attention to the details: How variations in U.S. grass-fed cattle-feed supplementation and finishing date influence human health.* Frontiers in Sustainable Food Systems, 6, Article 851494. https://doi.org/10.3389/fsufs.2022.851494

33.van Vliet, S., Provenza, F. D., & Kronberg, S. L. (2021). *Health-promoting phytonutrients are higher in grass-fed meat and milk.* Frontiers in Sustainable Food Systems, 5, Article 555426. https://doi.org/10.3389/fsufs.2020.555426

34.Ponnampalam, E. N., Hopkins, D. L., & Jacobs, J. L. (2018). *Increasing omega-3 levels in meat from ruminants under pasture-based systems.* Revue Scientifique et Technique de l'Office International des Epizooties, 37(1), 267–280.

35.Memme, J. M., Erlich, A. T., Phukan, G., & Hood, D. A. (2021). Exercise and mitochondrial health. Journal of Physiology, 599(3), 803–817.

36.Park, S. Y., Gifford, J. R., Andtbacka, R. H. I., Trinity, J. D., Hyngstrom, J. R., Garten, R. S., Diakos, N. A., Ives, S. J., Dela, F., Larsen, S., Drakos, S., & Richardson, R. S. (2014). *Cardiac, skeletal, and smooth muscle mitochondrial respiration: Are all mitochondria created equal?* American Journal of Physiology–Heart and Circulatory Physiology, 307(3), H346–H352.

37.Suomalainen, A., & Nunnari, J. (2024). *Mitochondria at the crossroads of health and disease.* Cell, 187(11), 2601–2627. https://doi.org/10.1016/j.cell.2024.04.037

38.Ruiz, L. M., Libedinsky, A., & Elorza, A. A. (2021). *Role of copper on mitochondrial function and metabolism.* Frontiers in Molecular Biosciences, 8, Article 711227.

39.Baker, Z. N., Cobine, P. A., & Leary, S. C. (2017). The mitochondrion: a central architect of copper homeostasis. Metallomics : integrated biometal science, 9(11), 1501–1512. https://doi.org/10.1039/c7mt00221a

40.Pizzorno, J. M. (2014, April). Mitochondria—Fundamental to life and health. Integrative Medicine: A Clinician's Journal, 13(2), 8–15. PMID: 26770084; PMCID: PMC4684129

41.Allen, J., Romay-Tallon, R., Brymer, K. J., Caruncho, H. J., & Kalynchuk, L. E. (2018). Mitochondria and mood: Mitochondrial dysfunction as a key player in the manifestation of depression. Frontiers in Neuroscience, 12, Article 386. https://doi.org/10.3389/fnins.2018.00386

42.San-Millán I. (2023). The Key Role of Mitochondrial Function in Health and Disease. Antioxidants (Basel, Switzerland), 12(4), 782.

43.Chen, W., Zhao, H., & Li, Y. (2023). Mitochondrial dynamics in health and disease: Mechanisms and potential targets. Signal Transduction and Targeted Therapy, 8, Article 333.

44.Kochanek, K. D., Xu, J. Q., & Arias, E. (2020). Mortality in the United States, 2019 (NCHS Data Brief No. 395). Hyattsville, MD: National Center for Health Statistics.

NOTES:

45.Myhill, S. (2018). *Diagnosis and treatment of chronic fatigue syndrome and myalgic encephalitis: It's mitochondria, not hypochondria.* Hammersmith Books.
46.Singh, P., Kaushik, U., Mir, S. R., Kukreti, N., & Visht, S. (2025). *Dietary and nutritional aspects of metabolic syndrome management: An overview.* Endocrine, Metabolic & Immune Disorders - Drug Targets. https://doi.org/10.2174/0118715303316445241108100017
47.Asim, M., Sajjad, M., Fatima, M., Zahid, A. H., Nasir, N. U. A., Alam, I., ... & Ishfaq, H. (2025). *The role of dietary interventions in improving gut microbiota and overall health.* International Journal of Research and Innovation in Social Science.
48.Garnås, E. (2023). *Fermented vegetables as a potential treatment for irritable bowel syndrome.* Current Developments in Nutrition, 7(2), 100039.
49.Mehboob, R. (2023). *Gut microbiome and digestive health.* Pakistan Journal of Health Sciences, 4(12).
50.Leeuwendaal, N. K., Stanton, C., O'Toole, P. W., & Beresford, T. P. (2022). *Fermented foods, health and the gut microbiome.* Nutrients, 14(7), 1527.
51.Bell, V., Ferrão, J., Pimentel, L. L., Pintado, M., & Fernandes, T. (2018). *One health, fermented foods, and gut microbiota.* Foods, 7(12), 195.
52.Buss, C., Kraemer-Aguiar, L. G., Maranhão, P. A., Marinho, C., Coelho de Souza, M. G., Wiernsperger, N., & Bouskela, E. (2012). Novel findings in the cephalic phase of digestion: A role for microcirculation? Physiology & Behavior, 105(4), 1082–1089. .
53.Uneyama, H., Tanaka, T., & Torii, K. (2004). Gut nutrient sensing by the abdominal vagus. Folia Pharmacologica Japonica, 124(4), 210–216.
54.de Waal, D. (2018). Digestion and absorption. In Nephrolithiasis: Basic, Diagnostic and Treatment Concepts (pp. 53–66). Springer.
55.Keller, J. (2013). Gastrointestinal digestion and absorption. In Encyclopedia of Human Nutrition (3rd ed.).
56.McCarthy, H. (2019). How to retrain your appetite: Lose weight permanently eating all your favourite foods. Pavilion Books (Collins & Brown). ISBN 978-1-911624-47-9
57.Mazza, E., Troiano, E., Ferro, Y., Lisso, F., Tosi, M., Lo Turco, E. G., Pujia, R., & Montalcini, T. (2024). *Obesity, dietary patterns, and hormonal balance modulation: Gender-specific impacts.* Nutrients, 16(11), 1629.
58.Trindade, F. (2020). *Nutritional influences on hormonal health.* In Integrative and Functional Medical Nutrition Therapy (pp. 633–647). Springer.
59.Velmurugan, G.*, Colella, M., & Santacroce, L. (2024).* Editorial: Endocrine disruptors in gut endocrinology. Frontiers in Endocrinology.
60.Topalović, O. (2022). Endocrine disruption and male reproductive health. In Endocrine Disruption and Human Health (pp. 137–152). Elsevier.
61.Hugara, S., Bala, S., & Gaja, J. B. (2024). A short survey for understanding hormonal imbalance and its causes. International Journal of Research and Review, 11(4).
62.Panda, C. S., Komarnytsky, S., Marsh, C. J., Barron, K. A., Le Brun-Blashka, S., & Metzger, B. T. (2023). Guided metabolic detoxification program supports Phase II detoxification enzymes and antioxidant balance in healthy participants. Nutrients, 15(9), 2209.
63.Cline, J. C. (2015). Nutritional aspects of detoxification in clinical practice. Alternative Therapies in Health and Medicine.

NOTES:

64.Walters, D. G., Young, P. J., Agus, C., Knize, M. G., Boobis, A. R., Gooderham, N. J., & Lake, B. G. (2004). *Cruciferous vegetable consumption alters the metabolism of the dietary carcinogen PhIP in humans.* Carcinogenesis, 25(9), 1657–1664.
65.Leoncini, E., Malaguti, M., Angeloni, C., Motori, E., Fabbri, D., & Hrelia, S. (2011). *Sulforaphane affects Phase II enzyme expression in cardiomyocytes through Akt signaling*. Journal of Food Science, 76(7), H182–H188.
66.Popova, L. D., Vasylyeva, I. M., & Nakonechna, O. A. (2021). *Correlation differences between sex and stress hormones in men and women.* Journal of Medicine and Biology Studies, 6(1), 327–335.
67.Soules, M. R., Merriggiola, M. C., Steiner, R. A., Clifton, D. K., Toivola, B., & Bremner, W. J. (1994). *Short-term fasting in normal women: Absence of effects on gonadotrophin secretion and the menstrual cycle*. Clinical Endocrinology, 40(6), 725–731.
66.Cienfuegos, S., et al. (2022). *Effect of intermittent fasting on reproductive hormone levels in females and males: A review of human trials.* Nutrients, 14(11), 2343.
http://doi.org./10.3390/nu14112343
67.Gabel, K., Hoddy, K. K., Haggerty, N., Song, J., Kroeger, C. M., Trepanowski, J. F., Panda, S., & Varady, K. A. (2018). *Effects of 8-hour time-restricted feeding on body weight and metabolic disease risk factors in obese adults: A pilot study.* Nutrition and Healthy Aging, 4(4), 345–353.
68.Tinsley, G. M., & La Bounty, P. M. (2015). *Effects of intermittent fasting on body composition and clinical health markers in humans.* Nutrition Reviews, 73(10), 661–674.
69.Pelz, M. (2022). *Fast like a girl: A woman's guide to using the healing power of fasting to burn fat, boost energy, and balance hormones.* Hay House, Incorporated.
70.Pelz, M. (2023). *The menopause reset: Get rid of your symptoms and feel like your younger self again.* Hay House, Incorporated

Chapter 5: Movement

1.Oral, O. (2024). *The role of physical activity on women's health*. Endocrinology and Disorders: Open Access, 8(1), 170.
2.Benini, R., Pr Nunes, P., Orsatti, C. L., Barcelos, L. C., & Orsatti, F. L. (2015). *Effects of acute total body resistance exercise on hormonal and cytokine changes in men and women.* Journal of Sports Medicine and Physical Fitness, 55(4), 363–370.
3.McTiernan, A., Sorensen, B., Irwin, M. L., Morgan, A., Yasui, Y., Rudolph, R. E., ... & Potter, J. D. (2007). *Exercise effect on weight and body fat in men and women.* Obesity, 15(6), 1496–1512. https://doi.org/10.1038/oby.2007.178
4.Balpande, M., & Siddiqui, S. (2022). *Effect of walking exercise on the human body.* International Journal of Health Sciences, 6(S1), 6977.https://doi.org/10.53730/ijhs.v6ns1.6977
5.Reynolds, A. N., Mann, J., Williams, S. M., & Venn, B. J. (2016). *Advice to walk after meals is more effective for lowering postprandial glycaemia in type 2 diabetes mellitus than advice that does not specify timing: a randomised crossover study*. Diabetologia, 59(12), 2572–2578. https://doi.org/10.1007/S00125-016-4085-2
6.Song, B., & Thomas, D. M. (2006). Dynamics of starvation in humans. Journal of Mathematical Biology, 53(5), 693–710.
https://doi.org/10.1007/s00285-006-0037-7

NOTES:

7.Carlson, M. G., Snead, W. L., & Campbell, P. J. (1994). Fuel and energy metabolism in fasting humans. The American Journal of Clinical Nutrition, 60(1), 29–36. https://doi.org/10.1093/ajcn/60.1.29

8.Carey, D. G. (2009). *Quantifying differences in the "fat burning" zone and the aerobic zone: implications for training.* Journal of Strength and Conditioning Research, 23(10), 2680–2685. https://doi.org/10.1519/JSC.0B013E3181BAC5C5

9.Snow, M. G., Kaeferlein, B., & Thieret, J. G. (2001). *Method for detecting anaerobic threshold and prescribing a training zone to maximize fat utilization or improved cardiovascular fitness.* Patent US6325741B1.

10.McLellan, T. M., & Gass, G. C. (1989). *Metabolic and cardiorespiratory responses relative to the anaerobic threshold.* Medicine and Science in Sports and Exercise, 21(2), 191–198. https://doi.org/10.1249/00005768-198904000-00013

11.Scherr, J., Wolfarth, B., Christle, J. W., Pressler, A., Wagenpfeil, S., & Halle, M. (2013). *Associations between Borg's rating of perceived exertion and physiological measures of exercise intensity.* European Journal of Applied Physiology, 113(1), 147–155. https://doi.org/10.1007/S00421-012-2421-X

12.Svensson, P., Hellberg, M., Wisén, A., & Clyne, N. (2024). *The Borg scale—efficient and safe for exercise prescription in self-administered balance and strength exercise in patients with CKD.* Nephrology Dialysis Transplantation. https://doi.org/10.1093/ndt/gfae069.734

13.Hutchinson, M., Kouwijzer, I., de Groot, S., & Goosey-Tolfrey, V. L. (2021). Comparison of two Borg exertion scales for monitoring exercise intensity in able-bodied participants and those with paraplegia and tetraplegia. Spinal Cord, 59, 470–478. https://doi.org/10.1038/s41393-021-00642-4

Chapter 6: The Pause

1.Sleep, Circadian Rhythm & Human Health
Walker, M. (2017). Why we sleep: Unlocking the power of sleep and dreams. Scribner.

2.Kim, H. O., Kang, I., Choe, W., & Yoon, K.-S. (2021). Sleep duration and risk of obesity: A genome and epidemiological study. World Academy of Science Journal, 3(2), 1–8.

3.Taporoski, T., Mead, M. P., & Knutson, K. L. (2023). Morbidity and mortality associated with sleep length. In K. L. Knutson (Ed.), Handbook of Clinical Neurology (Vol. 190, pp. 1391–1395). Elsevier.

4.Tubbs, A. S., Ghani, S. B., Valencia, D., Jean-Louis, G., Killgore, W. D. S., Fernandez, F.-X., & Grandner, M. A. (2022). Racial/ethnic minorities have greater declines in sleep duration with higher risk of cardiometabolic disease: An analysis of the U.S. National Health Interview Survey. Sleep Epidemiology, 2, 100022.

5.Schmid, S. M., Hallschmid, M., Jauch-Chara, K., Born, J., & Schultes, B. (2008). *A single night of sleep deprivation increases ghrelin levels and feelings of hunger in normal-weight healthy men.* Journal of Sleep Research, 17(3), 331–334.

6.Borges, C. M. (2018). Is there a relationship between sleep and obesity? Endocrinology & Metabolism International Journal, 6(3), 191.

7.Rahman, S. A., Grant, L. K., Cohn, A., Nathan, M., Harder, J., Gonsalvez, I., ... & Joffe, H. (2023). *Impact of sleep fragmentation and estradiol suppression on leptin, ghrelin, satiety and hunger in women: An experimental menopause mode*l. Journal of the Endocrine Society, 7(Supplement_1), bvad114.020.

NOTES:

8.Grzelak, A. (2024). Managing blue light exposure: *Impacts on sleep quality and circadian health.* Quality in Sport, 25, Article 56741. https://doi.org/10.12775/qs.2024.25.56741
9.Vethe, D., Scott, J., Engström, M., Salvesen, Ø., Sand, T., Olsen, A., ... & Kallestad, H. (2021). *The evening light environment in hospitals can be designed to produce less disruptive effects on the circadian system and improve sleep*. Sleep, 44(3), zsaa194. https://doi.org/10.1093/sleep/zsaa194
10.Hidayat, M. T., Nurmaulid, A., Wulandari, D. S., Muto'an, A. S., & Aditya, D. (2023). *Light wavelength exposure and sleep quality in young adults.* Bhinneka, 2(1). http://doi.rog/10.59024/bhineka.v2i1.621
11.Yeom, J. W., & Cho, C.-H. (2024). *Herbal and natural supplements for improving sleep: A literature review.* Psychiatry Investigation, 21(8), Article e0121. http://doi.org/10.30773/pi.2024.0121
12.Lakhan, S. E., & Finesmith, R. B. (2013). *Nutritional supplements and sleep: An overview.* In Nutrition and Functional Foods for Healthy Aging (pp. 547–563). Wageningen Academic Publishers. http://doi.org/10.3920/9789086867639_028
13.Chabo, A., & Srivastava, S. B. (2024). Catching ZZZs: *A summary of the most common herbal medications taken for insomnia.* American Journal of Lifestyle Medicine. http://doi.org/10.1177/15598276241232953
14.Light Exposure, Circadian Rhythm & Environmental Misalignment
VoPham, T., Ton, M., & Weaver, M. D. (2024). Spatiotemporal light exposure modeling for environmental circadian misalignment and solar jetlag. Environmental Epidemiology, 25, Article e0301.
15.Kok, E. Y., Kaur, S., Shukri, N. H. M., Razak, N. A., Takahashi, M., Teoh, S. C., Tay, J. E. F., & Shibata, S. (2024). The role of light exposure in infant circadian rhythm establishment: A scoping review perspective. European Journal of Pediatrics, 183(12).
16.Tähtämö, L., Partonen, T., & Pesonen, A.-K. (2019). Systematic review of light exposure impact on human circadian rhythm. Chronobiology International, 36(2), 151–170.
17. Precedence Research. *Health and wellness market size, trends, growth.* Precedence Research, 2024, https://www.precedenceresearch.com/health-and-wellness-market. Accessed 29 July 2025.
18.U.S. Congress. (2023). *Consolidated Appropriations Act, 2024.* Public Law No. 117–328.
19.U.S. Congress. (2010). *Patient Protection and Affordable Care Act*, Pub. L. No. 111–148, 124 Stat. 119.

Chapter 7: The Jesus Way

1.Zec, M. M., et al. (2023). *A single 36-h water-only fast vastly remodels the plasma lipidome.* Frontiers in Cardiovascular Medicine, 10, 1251122.
2.Vohra, P., & Jasuja, K. (2016). *15 days 'water only fast': A tough but a challenging personal experience.* International Journal of Scientific Reports, 2(9).
3.Mackieh, R., et al. (2023).*Unlocking the benefits of fasting: A review of its impact on various biological systems and human health.* Current Medicinal Chemistry, 30(27), 327549.
4.Reddy, B. L., et al. (2024). *Health benefits of intermittent fasting*. Repository.

NOTES:

5.Menigoz, W., Latz, T. T., Ely, R. A., Kamei, C., Melvin, G., & Sinatra, D. (2020). *Integrative and lifestyle medicine strategies should include Earthing (grounding): Review of research evidence and clinical observations.* Explore, 16(3), 152–160.
https://doi.org/10.1016/j.explore.2019.10.005
6.Oschman, J. L. (2022).*Illnesses in technologically advanced societies due to lack of grounding (Earthing).* Biomedical Journal, 45(6), 1061–1072. https://doi.org/10.1016/j.bj.2022.10.004
7.Koniver, L. (2024).*Grounding: An anti-aging breakthrough?* Unpublished Manuscript, https://doi.org/10.33425/2996-3893.1014
8.Grzelak, A. (2024).*Managing blue light exposure: Impacts on sleep quality and circadian health.* Quality in Sport, 25, Article 56741.
9.Swamy, D. A. (2023).Review on the study of potential health hazards caused by blue light due to melanopsin activity. International Journal of Advanced Chemical Research, 5(1), Article 146.
10.Alam, M., Abbas, K., Sharf, Y., & Khan, S. (2024).Impacts of blue light exposure from electronic devices on circadian rhythm and sleep disruption in adolescent and young adult students. Chronobiology in Medicine, 4(1), Article 0004.
11.Reign, D., Dailey, N. S., King, R., Grandner, M. A., Alkozei, A., & Killgore, W. D. S. (2022). 0037 Blue light exposure facilitates cortical neural efficiency exclusive of melatonin effects. Sleep, 45(Supplement_1), A15.

One Final Message

FROM MY HEART

YOU ARE ENOUGH

My prayer for you today is that you would know this deeply:

No matter what season you are in, no matter how your body feels, and no matter what your journey has looked like, you are enough.

God is not looking for perfect vessels. He is searching the world over for yielded vessels who will surrender their ways, their will, and their lives to Him.

In Isaiah 55:8–9, He reminds us:

"'For my thoughts are not your thoughts, neither are your ways my ways,' declares the Lord. 'As the heavens are higher than the earth, so are my ways higher than your ways and my thoughts than your thoughts.'"

God has a plan and a purpose for your life. If you are holding this book, it is not by accident. Your life matters in His grand story of redemption. He is writing a testimony through your life, even now.

Every person has a unique story, and that story has the power to change the world.

And when you feel weak, discouraged, or not enough,
remember this promise:

*"My grace is sufficient for you, for My strength
is made perfect in weakness."*

— 2 Corinthians 12:9

Keep walking.
Keep growing.
Keep surrendering.
God is not finished with you yet!

Believing God's BEST for you,

Staci

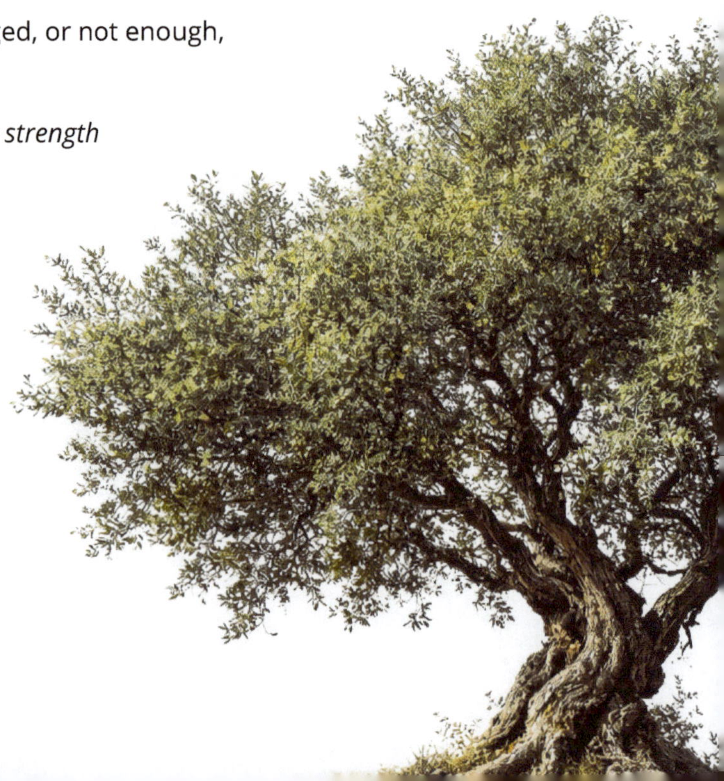

ABOUT THE AUTHOR

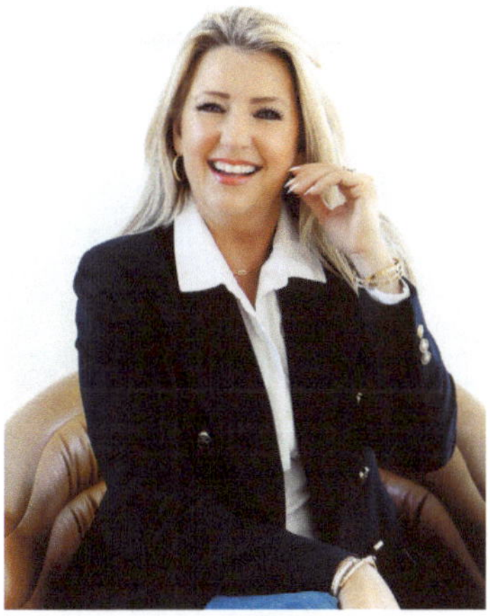

Staci Wallace is an 8x author, leadership strategist, international speaker, and founder of Fueled by Fire, a global movement helping Kingdom-minded leaders build lives and businesses of lasting impact without sacrificing faith, family, or freedom.

After four decades of coaching thousands of top leaders, Staci kept seeing the same pattern. The most accomplished people in the room were quietly exhausted, depleted, and far from whole. Most had been told that wellness meant better food choices, more steps, or a stricter fitness routine. What she discovered goes much deeper. The greater cause of sickness, disease, and depletion in the lives of high-performing leaders is not a lack of discipline. It is living outside of God's blueprint for wholeness, the integrated design of spirit, soul, and body that Scripture has always pointed to.

She and her husband, Larry, are the founders of Epiphany Ranch in East Texas, a gathering place for leaders pursuing Kingdom alignment in every area of life.

Her book, *Fueled*, is Staci's call to every leader to stop managing symptoms and start building the kind of wholeness God designed them for.

SPECIAL CONTRIBUTIONS

Irina Chifor, DipION, mBANT, rCNHC, is a certified nutritionist trained in the principles of functional medicine and holistic wellness. Through her clinical work with clients and leaders around the world, she helps individuals restore health by addressing the root causes of metabolic imbalance, inflammation, and hormone imbalance.

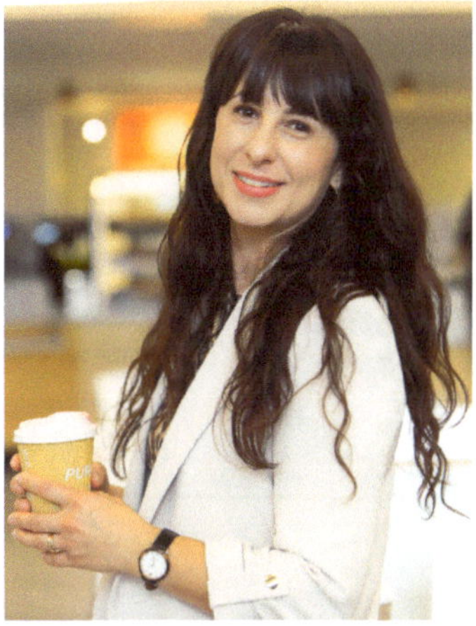

Her approach combines nutritional science, lifestyle optimization, and faith-centered wellness principles to support lasting transformation. Irina's expertise helped shape the nutritional and functional health insights found throughout Fueled.

FOR ADDITIONAL RESOURCES BY STACI WALLACE

Use your phone's camera to
scan this code:

or visit

WWW.STACIWALLACE.COM

www.ingramcontent.com/pod-product-compliance
Lightning Source LLC
LaVergne TN
LVHW070935210926
848482LV00003B/248

* 9 7 8 1 7 3 2 7 9 1 6 7 1 *